THE TRUTH ABOUT
ABUSE

THE TRUTH ABOUT ABUSE

MARK J. KITTLESON, PH.D.
Southern Illinois University
General Editor

WILLIAM KANE, PH.D.
University of New Mexico
Adviser

RICHELLE RENNEGARBE, PH.D.
McKendree College
Adviser

John Haley
Principal Author

Wendy Stein
Principal Author

Facts On File, Inc.

The Truth About Abuse

Facts On File, Inc.
132 West 31st Street
New York NY 10001

Library of Congress Cataloging-in-Publication Data

Haley, John, 1959–
    The truth about abuse / Mark J. Kittleson, general editor; William Kane, adviser; Richelle Rennegarbe, adviser; John Haley, principal author, Wendy Stein, principal author.
    p. cm.
    Includes index
    ISBN 0-8160-5297-2 (hc: alk. paper)
    1. Family violence. 2. Child abuse. 3. Older people—Abuse of. 4. Women—Abuse of. 5. Dating violence. 6. Psychological abuse. 7. Sex crimes. I. Kittleson, Mark J., 1952– II. Kane, William, 1947– III. Rennegarbe, Richelle. IV. Title.
    HV6625.H35 2005
    362.82′92—dc22   2004023157

Facts On File books are available at special discounts when purchased in bulk quantities for businesses, associations, institutions, or sales promotions. Please call our Special Sales Department in New York at (212) 967-8800 or (800) 322-8755.

You can find Facts On File on the World Wide Web at http://www.factsonfile.com

Text design by David Strelecky
Cover design by Cathy Rincon
Graphs by Sholto Ainslie

Printed in the United States of America

MP Hermitage 10 9 8 7 6 5 4 3 2

This book is printed on acid-free paper.

CONTENTS

LIST OF
ILLUSTRATIONS
AND TABLES

PREFACE

In developing The Truth About series, we have taken time to review some of the most pressing problems facing our youths today. Issues such as alcohol and drug abuse, depression, family problems, sexual activity, and eating disorders are at the top of a list of growing concerns. It is the intent of these books to provide vital facts while also dispelling myths about these terribly important and all-too-common situations. These are authoritative resources that kids can turn to in order to get an accurate answer to a specific question or to research the history of a problem, giving them access to the most current related data available. It is also a reference for parents, teachers, counselors, and others who work with youths and require detailed information.

Let's take a brief look at the issues associated with each of those topics. Alcohol and drug use and abuse continue to be a national concern. Today's young people often use drugs to avoid life's extraordinary pressures. In doing so they are losing their ability to learn how to cope effectively. Without the internal resources to cope with pressure, adolescents turn increasingly back to addictive behaviors. As a result, the problems and solutions are interrelated. Also, the speed with which the family structure is changing often leaves kids with no outlet for stress and no access to support mechanisms.

In addition, a world of youths faces the toughest years of their lives, dealing with the strong physiological urges that accompany sexual desire. Only when young people are presented the facts honestly, without indoctrination, are they likely to connect risk taking with certain behaviors. This reference set relies on knowledge as the most important tool in research and education.

Finally, one of the most puzzling issues of our times is that of eating disorders. Paradoxically, while our youths are obsessed with thinness and beauty and go to extremes to try to meet perceived societal expectations, they are also increasingly plagued by obesity. Here, too, separating the facts from fiction is an important tool in research and learning.

As much as possible, The Truth About presents the facts through honest discussions and reports of the most up-to-date research. Knowing the facts associated with health-related questions and problems will help young people make informed decisions in school and throughout life.

Mark J. Kittleson, Ph.D.
General Editor

HOW TO USE THIS BOOK

NOTE TO STUDENTS

Knowledge is power. By possessing knowledge you have the ability to make decisions, ask follow-up questions, or know where to go to obtain more information. In the world of health, that is power! That is the purpose of this book—to provide you the power you need to obtain unbiased, accurate information and *The Truth About Abuse.*

Topics in each volume of The Truth About are arranged in alphabetical order, from A to Z. Each of these entries defines its topic and explains in detail the particular issue. At the end of most entries are cross-references to related topics. A list of all topics by letter can be found in the table of contents or at the back of the book in the index.

How have these books been compiled? First, the publisher worked with me to identify some of the country's leading authorities on key issues in health education. These individuals were asked to identify some of the major concerns that young people have about such topics. The writers read the literature, spoke with health experts, and incorporated their own life and professional experiences to pull together the most up-to-date information on health issues, particularly those of interest to adolescents and of concern in *Healthy People 2010.*

Throughout the alphabetical entries, the reader will find sidebars that separate Fact from Fiction. There are Question-and-Answer boxes that attempt to address the most common questions that youth ask about sensitive topics. In addition, readers will find special features called "Teens Speak"—case studies of teens with personal stories related to the topic in hand.

This may be one of the most important books you will ever read. Please share it with your friends, families, teachers, and classmates. Remember, you possess the power to control your future. One way to affect your course is through the acquisition of knowledge. Good luck and keep healthy.

NOTE TO LIBRARIANS

This book, along with the rest of The Truth About series, serves as a wonderful resource for young researchers. It contains a variety of facts, case studies, and further readings that the reader can use to help answer questions, formulate new questions, or determine where to go to find more information. Even though the topics may be considered delicate by some, don't be afraid to ask patrons if they have questions. Feel free to direct them to the appropriate sources, but do not press them if you encounter reluctance. The best we can do as educators is to let young people know that we are there when they need us.

Mark J. Kittleson, Ph.D.
General Editor

ABUSIVE BEHAVIOR

Abuse is a pattern of behavior used to control another person. The behavior can be physical, emotional, verbal, social, or sexual. Abuse does not always result in broken bones, black eyes, or cuts and bruises. Nonphysical abuse can break a person's spirit and shatter his or her confidence and self-esteem.

Tragically, it is at home—where a person is supposed to feel safe and loved—that most abuse occurs. For many people, home and family do not provide the "warm and fuzzy" feelings that television ads and sitcoms portray. Instead, home can be a place filled with anger, yelling, insults, sexual violence, beatings, and even killings. Americans are more likely to be beaten or assaulted at home than on the street. Americans are also more likely to be hurt by the people they know—and love—than by strangers.

Every year, millions of people suffer some form of abuse at the hands of friends, relatives, and other loved ones. Elderly parents are beaten by their adult children, other relatives, or in-home caregivers. Children are abused and neglected by parents. Teenagers become involved in dangerous dating relationships. In 1999, the *Journal of the American Medical Association* reported that physical violence occurs in four to six million intimate relationships every year. The same year, an article in *Archives of Neurology* titled "Domestic Violence in Neurologic Practice" estimated that 25 percent of all women in the United States will be abused during their lifetimes. Males commit the overwhelming majority of these attacks. According to the Bureau of Justice Statistics's (BJS) 2000 report *Intimate Partner Violence*, men commit over 80 percent of these assaults.

Amazingly, many victims fail to even recognize their treatment as abuse. They may know something is wrong. They may know that they do not like how they are treated. However, they have never looked at their treatment for what it is—violent and even criminal behavior. In the 2002 essay "Domestic Violence and the Criminal Justice System: An Overview," the *Online Journal of Issues in Nursing* pointed out that, until the 1960s, the police generally considered domestic violence a private matter. Arrests for domestic violence, a **misdemeanor**, were very rare, and the general attitude was that such matters should be handled by the family, not the police.

TYPES OF ABUSE

In this book, we will look at many forms of abuse, including the abuse of domestic partners, the elderly, dates, children, parents, and siblings. Within each of these types of abuse, there are many forms of abusive behavior.

Physical abuse

Physical abuse is the use of strength or weapons or the threat of injury to hurt or control another person. Physical abuse ranges from pushing to murder. Many types of physical abuse are crimes; those committed by relatives or domestic partners are rarely reported to the police. Relatives and domestic partners often are reluctant to file criminal charges against a loved one. *Intimate Partner Violence* found that only half of white female abuse victims and about two-thirds of black and Hispanic victims reported abuse to the police.

Physically abusive behavior includes:

- Throwing or breaking things, punching walls, or tearing clothes
- Grabbing, pushing, shoving, shaking, hitting, slapping, biting, pinching, hair-pulling, arm-twisting, or spitting
- Withholding food, clothing, sleep, or medicine
- Keeping a person locked up
- Abusing animals
- Using weapons or threats of using a weapon
- Causing broken bones or internal injuries

- Abandoning a person in a dangerous place
- Failing to take care of a person you are supposed to care for (child, elderly person, or sick or helpless partner)

Emotional and verbal abuse

Emotional abuse is the use of words and actions to control or hurt another person. Although common, emotional abuse is harder to identify than physical abuse. It is not recognized as criminal unless it involves a serious physical threat. Despite the claim of the old nursery rhyme, "Sticks and stones may break my bones, but names will never hurt me," names do hurt. Emotional abuse can inflict injuries that last a lifetime—long after physical wounds heal.

Many families simply accept emotional abuse as normal. After all, don't most couples fight? Don't most parents yell at their kids? And don't most people get frustrated and say things they shouldn't? Emotional abuse, however, involves repeated hurtful words or acts that disregard the other person's feelings. Unfortunately, these hurtful behaviors can become "normal" communication within a family. The targets of the abuse become emotionally damaged and don't even know why they feel so badly about themselves and their world.

Emotionally abusive behavior includes words and actions. Types of verbal abuse include:

- Insults, put-downs and name-calling (for example, saying a person is stupid or ugly, or calling someone a liar)
- Threats to harm you or someone you love
- Yelling
- Sarcasm
- Constant criticism
- Leaving nasty messages on an answering machine
- Sending cruel letters or e-mails
- False or malicious accusations
- Sending mixed signals

Emotionally abusive behaviors include:

- Controlling all finances or major decisions
- Isolating the other person from friends or family members

- Blackmail or threats to reveal one's sexual orientation or other sensitive information
- Using lies to manipulate
- Making faces
- Making another person economically dependent
- Threatening to commit suicide if abandoned
- Threatening to kill a partner who attempts to leave
- Constantly questioning one's partner about his or her activities
- Taking or destroying possessions
- Humiliation (for example, making accusations in front of others or making a person do something embarrassing)

Sexual abuse

Sexual abuse involves using sexual behavior as a way to control the actions or behaviors of another person. Thus, sexual abuse is not primarily a sexual act; it is first and foremost an act of control. Children and adults, males and females, are sexually abused. When sexual abuse occurs between partners or people who are dating, it is meant to exert power and to humiliate. Sexually abusive behavior includes:

- Sexual jokes or demeaning remarks toward your sex
- Name-calling involving sexual language
- Demands for sex
- Unwanted touching
- Demanding sex by using threats
- Withholding sex as punishment
- False accusations of unfaithfulness
- Rape

WHO IS INVOLVED IN ABUSE?

Batterers and their victims come from all walks of life, but researchers have identified some general characteristics of both abusers and the targets of their abuse. These characteristics cannot predict whether someone will be a perpetrator or victim of abuse. They can, however, alert people to the danger and help possible victims as well as potential batterers recognize danger signs in their own behavior and seek professional help.

Victims of abuse typically have low self-esteem. They often are unsure of their own needs and often tend to define themselves in terms of their spouse, children, or family. Their partners use criticism and put-downs to maintain emotional control over the victims who come to believe that they deserve to be treated poorly.

Targets of abuse tend to blame themselves for the mistreatment they endure. They may think that they provoke their partners' anger or tell themselves that the abuser can't help his or her actions. Victims frequently blame themselves for not doing enough to make their abusers change.

Although abused domestic partners constantly blame themselves for not doing enough to make things right, they are somewhat passive in the face of abuse. They put up with great emotional distress and brutal beatings and still remain in the relationships. Victims may cling to the hope that the abuser's behavior will change, despite little or no evidence of improvement. They may feel that, somehow, everything will work itself out if they are just patient enough.

Victims of abuse often deny or minimize the abuse they suffer. Denial is a powerful survival tool. Targets of abuse may turn off their feelings to minimize the emotional damage from an abusive situation. They either deny that the abuse is occurring or make excuses for their abusers. They may even deny that they are being beaten. They convince themselves that they were just clumsy, that their injuries are the result of an accident, or that the abuser didn't really mean any harm.

Batterers believe that violence is acceptable. In many cases they learned this lesson in their childhood homes. According to the 1995 report "Characteristics of Batterers in a Multisite Evaluation of Batterer Interaction Systems," published by the Minnesota Center Against Violence and Abuse, 33 percent of males who abused their spouses grew up in homes marked by similar abuse, and 26 percent reported having been physically harmed by their parents. As children, they learned the language of abuse. They learned that violence was a way to get what they wanted, and they took this lesson with them into adulthood.

Unlike their victims, many abusers refuse to take responsibility for their behavior. They tend to blame their victims, claiming that some action or attitude by the victim led to the abuse. They may even deny that they caused an injury.

Abusers tend to become jealous of any other relationship their partners have, even those with friends or family. Those other relationships are seen as taking time and attention away from the abusers. Abusers have a need to control and overpower their partners, which is really a way of expressing fears that they will be abandoned. Abusers isolate their partners out of jealousy, which tends to make the partner more emotionally dependent. The more dependent the abused partners are, the more likely they are to feel that they can't make it on their own.

Parents and abuse
Parents, especially mothers, are responsible for most cases of child abuse and neglect in the United States. According to the U.S. Department of Health and Human Services, mothers perpetrated 40.3 percent of all child abuse violations in 2002, and mothers and fathers together committed an additional 18 percent. The World Health Organization (WHO) 2002 *World Report on Violence and Health* found that child abusers are likely to be young, single, poor, and unemployed. According to WHO, single mothers in the United States are three times more likely to physically punish their children than mothers in two-parent families.

Child abusers often suffer from an inability to control their impulses or deal with frustrations. This can lead to violent explosions of temper if they are frustrated by something a child says or does. WHO suggests that many people who commit child abuse are simply ill-informed about effective parenting strategies. They do not understand the needs of children at different stages of development. When their parenting strategies fail, they may boil over from frustration, anger, and self-criticism, and lash out at their children.

Like adult targets of abuse, abused children often suffer from low self-esteem and blame themselves for their abusers' behavior. Children who are abused are more likely to see violence as a way to settle disputes, and as adults they are more likely to abuse their own children. Children and adults often need counseling to let go of the notion that they somehow caused the abuse and even deserved it.

Abuse at school
Abuse is primarily about power and control. Most frequently, it occurs between people in dating or domestic relationships, but these are not the only settings in which abuse can occur. Abuse at school can be

just as damaging physically or emotionally as abuse suffered in a family or intimate relationship.

Take a look around your school. Abuse is not always something that happens out of view. Listen to the put-downs and insults in the hallways. You may be surprised at the abuse that takes place right in front of you. Does your school have a bully or a group of kids who pick on younger kids? Have you witnessed gay bashing in the hallways? Have you overheard remarks like "You're stupid," "You don't belong here," or "We don't want you at our table?" These are all examples of abusive behavior. If kids at school are posting lies and gossip on a Website, starting vicious rumors about another student, that, too, is abuse. Maybe you've heard about athletes or members of clubs who have had to perform humiliating deeds in order to be accepted. That is hazing, which is yet another form of abuse. If a teacher or other adult pressures you to have sex or threatens you if you don't, he or she is committing **sexual harassment**, a form of abuse.

People who are targets of abuse, whether at home or school, often live in fear and shame. They do not have to become lifelong victims, however. They need friends to stand by them and to help them get help. Reaching out to a teen who is being abused can help break the cycle of violence in which today's abused children become tomorrow's abusive parents.

RISKY BUSINESS SELF-TESTS

The following tests are designed to let you find out more about your own risk of becoming a victim or perpetrator of dating abuse. The first test focuses on your chances of becoming a target for dating abuse, a serious issue that many teens are too embarrassed or afraid to discuss. The second helps you assess whether you are actually in an abusive dating relationship. Keep a record of your answers on a separate piece of paper.

Could you be a target of dating abuse?

Answer "true" or "false" to these questions to assess whether you are or could be a target for dating abuse.

_____ I believe it is okay for my friends to run my life.

_____ I like it when someone makes decisions for me.

_____ I sometimes drink too much.

_____ I sometimes use drugs.

_____ I have been in an abusive relationship in the past.

_____ I drink and abuse drugs with people I don't know well.

_____ I sometimes say "Yes" when I don't really mean it.

_____ My parents are sometimes physically abusive to each other.

_____ My parents are emotionally abusive to each other.

_____ My parents physically abuse my siblings or me.

_____ My parents emotionally abuse my siblings or me.

_____ Many people in my family get into fights with each other.

_____ I am sometimes afraid of the person I am dating.

_____ I am afraid to talk honestly with my boyfriend/ girlfriend.

_____ I do not see my friends very often once I start a new relationship.

_____ I don't have a lot of confidence.

The person I am involved with:

_____ is jealous and possessive

_____ loses his/her temper often (has explosive outbursts)

_____ may have been abused as a child

_____ is cruel toward animals

_____ makes me feel guilty or humiliated

_____ tries to dominate me

_____ has few friends

_____ begs me not to leave

_____ threatens to kill himself/herself if I leave

_____ blames me for making him upset

_____ yells or hits me then brings me gifts and begs for forgiveness

_____ abuses drugs and/or alcohol

For each question to which you answered "true," your risk of being a target of dating or partner abuse now or in the future increases.

Could you be (or become) an abuser?

Answer "true" or "false" to these questions to assess whether you are or could be abusive in a dating or partner relationship.

_____ My boyfriend/girlfriend is afraid of me.

_____ I make most of the decisions in my relationship.

_____ I call or watch the actions of my boyfriend/girlfriend all the time to keep track of where he/she is.

_____ I have threatened to kill him/her.

_____ There is violence in my home.

_____ I have pushed or shoved my boyfriend/girlfriend.

_____ I often hurt his/her feelings with insults, name-calling or put-downs.

_____ I have intentionally broken things that my boyfriend/girlfriend owned.

_____ I think that I have a right to hit my boyfriend/girlfriend.

_____ I like to fool around with guns or knives.

_____ I have threatened to kill myself if he/she breaks up with me.

_____ My boyfriend/girlfriend makes me so mad I lose control.

[For males dating females:]

_____ I think my girlfriend should do what I say.

_____ I believe that guys should be tough and that showing emotion is a sign of weakness.

For each question to which you answer "True," your risk of being or becoming abusive toward a boyfriend, girlfriend, or partner increases.

A TO Z ENTRIES

■ ABUSE IN FAMILIES
See: Child Abuse; Domestic Partner Abuse

■ ABUSE IN SOCIETY
Social conditions and attitudes that allow the occurrence of patterns of behavior used to control other people. Americans live in a violent society. The news media, movies, and video games show strangers attacking people on the streets and in their homes. Sadly, people close to the victims commit much of the violence in communities through acts such as spousal abuse, child abuse, and elder abuse. Abusers are hurting the people they say they love.

PERPETRATORS OF ABUSE
Abuse comes in many forms, and abusers come from all walks of life, economic classes, professions, and ethnic and racial groups. They can be male, female, straight, bisexual, or gay. However, according to the Bureau of Justice Statistics (BJS), most **domestic partner** abuse is committed by men against women. The BJS 2000 report *Intimate Partner Violence* found that men are responsible for over 80 percent of all domestic abuse.

People who abuse their partners typically have low self-esteem and often believe they have failed to achieve important career or personal goals. These feelings of inadequacy may lead them to fear that their partners will stop loving them and abandon them. As a result, abusers try to control their partners through physical violence, **emotional abuse**, and/or financial dependence.

By contrast, women are responsible for most cases of child abuse (the use of physical, emotional, or verbal abuse to control the behavior of a child). According to the BJS a child's mother is more likely than any other person to be involved in abusing the child. The BJS reported in 2002 that in over 40 percent of child abuse cases in the United States, the child's mother was the sole perpetrator. In another 23 percent of the cases, the mother was accompanied by another abuser. The World Health Organization's 2000 *World Report on Violence and Health* found that parents who were young, single, poor, and/or unemployed were at greater risk for becoming child abusers.

The BJS reported that single mothers accounted for more child abuse than any other group in 2002.

HISTORY OF DOMESTIC ABUSE

Most societies throughout history have been **patriarchal**, meaning that the father or husband controlled power within the family. Males exerted control outside the home as well, dominating political, economic, and social power. Women had little or no power and few rights or privileges. For example, in ancient Rome a woman was subject to her father's rule until she married, then she was subject to the rule of her husband. If she left her husband, she had no rights to property or her children. Roman women could be beaten, divorced, and even killed for the same behaviors in which men routinely engaged— adultery, public drunkenness, or attending public games.

The tradition of male dominance is a part of Christian and Jewish religious writing, including the Bible. Some religious thinkers believe that Eve and all women were punished for eating the forbidden apple, while Adam and all men were given rule over women. A number of religious groups have supported this idea of male rule over women and even encouraged husbands to beat their wives as punishment for offenses. Some countries made minimal efforts to limit the scope of such beatings. For example, British law of the 1700s said that husbands had the right to "physically chastise" their wives as long as the stick they used was no thicker than their thumb. That is the basis for the saying "rule of thumb."

When English colonists settled in North America they brought their laws with them, including the right of a husband to beat his wife. Until recently, American courts preferred not to interfere with what happened between a husband and wife in the home. Domestic abuse was considered a private matter—not one in which the courts should become involved. As a result, husbands largely were free to deal with their wives as they chose until the late 1800s, when some states began to do away with laws that permitted wife beating. The "rule of thumb" was not overturned in Alabama or Massachusetts until 1871. In 1883 Maryland became the first state to outlaw wife beating.

Despite changes in the law, the individual's right to privacy and the sacredness of the home remained effective barriers to police intervention well into the 20th century. According to a 2002 article in the *Online Journal of Issues in Nursing* titled "Domestic Violence and the Criminal Justice System: An Overview," most police did not consider domestic violence to be a "real" crime. If the wife was not seriously hurt, the husband was rarely arrested or charged with a crime. Attitudes began to change with the coming of the women's movement in the 1970s. Activists demanded equal treatment for women, including stricter enforcement of the laws against domestic abuse. Today, state laws prosecute abusers and some states even provide funding for **battered** women shelters.

HISTORY OF CHILD ABUSE

Parents have traditionally held the same sort of power over their children as husbands have exerted over their wives. In some cases, the treatment of children has been even worse. Some societies have practiced **infanticide**, in which unwanted babies are abandoned to die of exposure or be killed by predators. A Roman father, for example, could refuse to accept a child for any reason. If he chose to do so, the child would be left to die.

According to a 2001 article in the journal *Family Matters* titled "A History of Child Protection Back to the Future? The Maltreatment of Children Has Occurred Throughout History," the use of physical force to punish children has long been accepted by many societies. Punishment was thought necessary in order to instill discipline and tame a child's naturally evil nature. This attitude prevailed in the United States almost unchallenged until the mid-1800s. In 1866 Henry Berge, founder of the Society for the Prevention of Cruelty to Animals, learned that a child was being mistreated by her foster parents. At the time, animals were protected from abuse but children were not. Berge argued to a court that the child was a member of the animal kingdom and therefore entitled to his group's protection. A judge agreed, and the case eventually led to the creation of the New York Society for the Prevention of Cruelty to Children. This was the first reported case of child abuse in the United States.

Fact Or Fiction?

The Bible says "Spare the rod and spoil the child."

Fact: The quote comes from the Book of Proverbs in the Bible. It has been used over and over again to justify **corporal punishment** (physical punishment) at home and school. The passage was originally written in Hebrew, and there are many different translations. According to the *New American Standard Bible*, the passage reads: "He who spares his rod hates his son, but he who loves him disciplines him diligently." That statement leaves room for much interpretation. Discipline means "to teach or guide." It is not a synonym for the word *punishment*. Also, a rod is not necessarily a stick used for beating; it can also refer to a symbol of power or authority.

In addition to being beaten, children were exploited as economic assets and sent to work at an early age. In agricultural societies even today, children work at home as soon as they are able to help with chores. However, until recently it was common for even very young children to work outside the home for strangers. The practice of apprenticeship, in which children were hired out to learn trades from master craftsmen, was widespread in Europe and North America until the 19th century. Child apprentices were subject to the same kinds of discipline from their masters as they received from their parents. However, maltreatment by strangers was treated differently from maltreatment by parents. In 1639 a man in Salem, Massachusetts, was tried for the death of his apprentice. Eight years later, another man was convicted of murdering his young servant. As punishment, the man's property was taken away and his hand burned. Nevertheless, parents were still free to abuse their own children—that was a family matter.

With the coming of the industrial age in the late 1700s, children began to work in factories. By the late 1800s, there were more than two million child workers in the United States. Children often worked the same hours as adults—12 hours a day, six days a week—in extremely dangerous conditions. Because working children were rarely able to attend school, most were illiterate. However, child labor was considered essential to the economic survival of many families. It was not until 1916 that the first law was passed in the United States to protect children in factories—the Keating-Owen Act. The United States did not outlaw child labor until 1938.

CULTURAL EXPECTATIONS

A pattern of abuse against women and children certainly exists. Thousands of years of viewing both groups as possessions has been hard to overcome. In addition, people still hold stereotypical views of male and female roles. Men are expected to be the breadwinners and to protect the family; women are expected to attend to the home and children. Men are supposed to be strong and silent and not show emotion; women are supposed to be more expressive, especially when it comes to their emotions. Men are seen as more coldly rational in decision making, while women are said to rely heavily on intuition. Although the definitions of what it means to be a man or woman are changing, these stereotypes are still used whenever people compare or judge the behaviors of men and women.

Popular media help to perpetuate these traditional views of women as less capable than men. A 1999 study reported in the journal *Sex Roles* found that male characters in television advertisements tend to be shown as tough, powerful, independent, successful, and knowledgeable. Women, on the other hand, were portrayed as young, thin, sexy, provocative, and available. The article, "Perpetuation of Subtle Prejudice: Race and Gender Imagery in 1990s Television Advertising," reported that women were typically shown in the home, while men were usually shown in work or outdoor situations. It also suggested that advertisers reinforce the idea of women as sex objects. White women in the advertisements routinely wore revealing clothing, tried to look pretty, or were being "checked out" by a man. Interestingly, the study found that African-American women were rarely portrayed as sex objects in television commercials.

Music videos and song lyrics have also come under fire for portraying women as sex objects or targets of abuse and physical violence. This charge is more frequently made against rap—particularly "gangsta" rap—than any other genre of popular music. In a 2001 article in the *Journal of Criminal Justice and Popular Culture*, researcher Edward G. Armstrong of Murray State University found that 22 percent of gangsta rap songs contained lyrics that degraded or advocated violence against women. The article goes so far as to suggest that the lyrics show evidence of a "rape culture" that devalues women and leads to violence against them.

Q & A

Question: What can I do when I hear put-downs about women and jokes about hitting them to make them "behave"?

Answer: If you hear these jokes and comments from people you know, you can say that they bother you. Point out that abuse is a big problem, especially to women. Your friends may accuse you of having no sense of humor, but they may think about what they say in front of you the next time. You may even find a few allies who will begin to intervene as well.

If you hear strangers or acquaintances making comments, think about whether saying something will cause the person to become violent. If so, perhaps you can take one person aside later and talk about your discomfort with the comments. You can also look for allies in the group who will support you if you speak out.

Despite evidence of some changes in attitudes toward domestic violence by law enforcement and the public at large, the image of the tough macho guy is still widely accepted. In many popular movies the hero kills the bad guys and "gets the girl" as his reward. The message is that being a man means being physically strong and willing to fight, while being a woman means waiting passively as the trophy for the strongest male.

Do the media messages about males, females, and how they treat one another reflect society's attitudes? Or are society's attitudes a result of these media messages? The situation is complex, and determining cause and effect is not simple. However, certain attitudes about the proper roles of men and women existed long before the invention of mass media such as radio, movies, and television. Nevertheless, the media have done little to discourage, and much to promote, the continued acceptance of gender stereotypes by society.

MORBIDITY AND MORTALITY

Morbidity is the rate of illness and injury among a population; mortality is the death rate among a population. As the following statistics reveal, morbidity and mortality due to domestic violence take a staggering toll in lives and health each year:

- According to the 2001 BJS report *Intimate Partner Violence and Age of Victim, 1993–1999*, more than three women a day in the United States are killed by their male partners.
- The BJS reports that there were 1,642 murders due to domestic violence in 1999, and 1,218 of the victims were women.
- The Federal Bureau of Investigation's *Uniform Crime Reports* for 1996 found that 30 percent of all female

murder victims in the United States were killed by their husbands or boyfriends.

■ According to the American Medical Association, one out of every three women treated in hospital emergency rooms are victims of violence. At least one in five has been injured by a current or former husband or boyfriend.

■ Three children each day die because of abuse or **neglect**, according to the U.S. Advisory Board on Child Abuse and Neglect. Children younger than one year accounted for 41 percent of child fatalities. Children younger than six years accounted for 85 percent of the fatalities.

■ Experts from the National Center for Prosecution of Child Abuse estimate that the number of child deaths from abuse and neglect could be as high as 5,000 annually.

The financial costs of abuse are also steep:

■ The American Medical Association journal *Medical News* claims that family violence costs the United States $5 billion to $10 billion each year. This total includes medical expenses as well as costs related to policing, courts, family shelters, foster care for children, sick leave, absenteeism, and lost productivity.

■ The *Puget Sound Business Journal* in 1998 quoted a study by Employee Assistance Providers that suggested 25 percent of workplace problems such as absenteeism, lower productivity, and excessive use of medical insurance are due to family violence.

■ Prevent Child Abuse America estimates that the United States spends $258 million a day on direct and indirect costs of child abuse and neglect. That works out to $94 billion a year. Of that figure, direct costs for hospitalization, mental health care, and treatment of chronic health problems are $26 million a day. Indirect costs include almost $13 million per day for health care, including care for mental health.

Society clearly has an important stake in fighting abuse. However, societal traditions and media messages frequently work to support rather than discredit the beliefs that make abuse possible and even acceptable. It is therefore up to individuals to make the choice to change their attitudes and reject messages that reinforce images of women and children as objects or property.

See also: Abusers, Common Traits of; Child Abuse; Domestic Partner Abuse; Homicide; Legal Intervention; Men and Abuse; Women and Abuse

FURTHER READING

Breiner, Sandra J. *Slaughter of the Innocents: Child Abuse through the Ages and Today.* New York: HarperCollins, 1990.
Dorne, Clifford K. *An Introduction to Child Maltreatment in the United States: History, Public Policy and Research, Third Edition.* Monsey, NY: Criminal Justice Press, 2002.
Pleck, Elizabeth. *Domestic Tyranny: The Making of American Social Policy against Family Violence from Colonial Times to the Present.* Champaign: University of Illinois Press, 2004.

■ ABUSE, THEORIES OF

Abuse is a complicated problem, and researchers have offered many different theories to explain it. Some of these theories seek explanations in the personality of the abuser. Others search for clues in the family environment. Still others look to the wider society for the causes of the problem. Determining the reasons abuse occurs is important because understanding a problem can help in prevention. The goal is to stop abuse from occurring in the first place.

TEENS SPEAK

I Grew Up with My Father Beating My Mother and Me

When I was little, I could hear the screaming from their room or from downstairs. As I got older, I finally understood what was going on. Sometimes months would go by and he didn't hurt her, but I always knew it was just a matter of time. Sometimes he was in such a rage, he would come after me with his belt, saying it was for my own good and that it was the only way I would learn to listen to him. Actually it was the way I learned what a loser he was. I learned to tune him out, not to listen to him.

When I was 14, I was bigger than him, and I thought I could stop him. I told him if he ever hit my mother or me again, I would kill him. I hated that I was even thinking that. The thing I wanted and still want most is to never be like him. He didn't like what I said either but for a different reason. He didn't like me telling him what to do. He said I was the kid and he was the father, and I would do as he said. He also didn't like that I was so close to my mother. I think he felt threatened that no matter how much power he thought he had, he couldn't control our love. The next time he went after my mother, I went after him. I was no match for him. He threw me against a wall and kicked me but at least it took the pressure off my mother.

Now I'm in college, and I still worry about my mother. She is still with him. I think that I will be okay because I have had a lot of support from a school counselor. My best friend's parents kind of "adopted me," and I got to see what a healthy family was like. It really helped to have other adults to turn to and good friends who understood and didn't judge my mother or me. I have good friends here at school too, and I have met others who also came from situations like mine. The school counseling center is even running a group for kids like me. I think it really helps to talk about it. I am afraid I could turn into a man like my dad, but I will work as hard as I can not to. I just hope that one of these days my mother will leave him for good.

PSYCHOLOGICAL THEORIES

Psychological theories of abuse look to factors inside the individual to explain abusive behavior. These factors include such things as personality, aggressiveness, and emotionality. There is considerable disagreement on the accuracy of psychological theories, but they still generate considerable research.

Psychoanalytic theory claims that abusers are insecure about their masculinity. In his 1985 article "Fighting for Control: A Clinical Assessment of Men Who Batter," psychiatrist Edward Gondolf argued that male abusers want to deny the feminine aspects of their personality, which they see as a source of weakness or shame. Abusers believe they can control the feminine aspects of their personalities by abusing women.

Personality theory looks at individual personality traits or characteristics for clues to the roots of abuse. For example, the 1991 study "Courtship Violence in a Canadian Sample of Male College Students" found that low self-esteem and high levels of anxiety characterized abusers. According to the 1984 publication *Temperament: Early Developing Personality Traits*, everyone has an inborn tendency to develop certain personality traits. This work was an outgrowth of earlier studies by psychologist Hans Eysenck, who argued that individual biology was an important factor in determining personality. According to these theories, abusers have certain inborn traits, including impulsiveness, anxiety, and an inability to feel empathy or sensitivity. While personality theory suggests that **heredity** is an important factor in abuse, not everyone who has inherited these personality traits will become an abuser.

Disinhibition theory focuses on the effect of alcohol on individual behavior as it relates to abuse. A 1997 study titled "The Role of Alcohol in Wife Beating and Child Abuse" suggests that alcohol lowers a person's inhibitions and releases violent impulses. The authors of the 1991 article "Personality, Alcohol Consumption, Alcohol Abuse and Male Perpetrated Spouse Abuse" cite evidence that certain persons are more prone than others to become violent and commit abuse when drinking.

Psychological theories of abuse have a great deal of intuitive appeal, but they suffer from several drawbacks. First of all, it can be difficult to determine whether a behavior is caused by internal or external factors because everyone grows up in slightly different circumstances. Therefore researchers cannot ensure that all of the abusers they are studying are operating under the same influences. Even if the researchers are reasonably sure that the cause of abuse is internal to an individual, they may find it difficult to figure out exactly which internal trait or traits are to blame. Not knowing the ultimate cause of the problem makes designing treatment or prevention programs problematic at best.

Q & A

Question: Does physical violence start right away in a relationship?

Answer: Abuse usually starts gradually and gets worse over time. It starts with insults and put-downs. The abuser begins to convince his partner that she needs to change because she is causing problems in the relationship. Then he expresses his jealousy and tries to isolate her from people or activities she cares about. He says he loves her so much that he doesn't want to be separated from her. The verbal abuse escalates, and he blames her for his own failures. She spends most of her energy and time catering to his emotional needs. She may even drink alcohol or take drugs with him because he insists. The hitting or other physical violence comes later, when she feels miserable about herself, and her confidence and self-image have been shattered. She may even believe she doesn't deserve to be happy.

FAMILY DYNAMICS THEORIES

The family dynamics approach argues that abuse is a problem that affects all family members, not just the abuser and the direct victims. Domestic violence is seen as the product of faulty family interactions. Family dynamics theories claim that family interactions can increase or decrease the likelihood of violence.

Psychologist Lenore Walker developed a theory called the cycle of violence that is a good example of a family systems approach. Walker says that in many abusive relationships, periods of abuse alternate with periods of relative peace. Her theory outlines a three-phase cycle of abusive behavior in which the actions of each partner play an important role in the pattern of abuse.

In the first phase, tension builds as the spouse becomes more moody and short-tempered. This phase is often followed by an explosion that may result in physical violence. Finally, in the "honeymoon" stage, the abuser apologizes and promises not to explode again. However, before long, the cycle starts all over again. According to Walker, the abused spouse develops **learned helplessness**, a condition in which the victim has been abused so often that she feels trapped and stops even trying to escape.

Family systems approaches have been criticized because of what some see as a bias against women. Feminists complain that these theories assign too much responsibility for violence to the actions of the female partner. For example, a 1990 article titled "Leveling, Civility and Violence in the Family" claimed that the way family members react to violence can create a "positive feedback loop" that reinforces the violence and allows it to continue and escalate. Critics see this kind of explanation as "blaming the victim," and they argue that such an attitude provides abusive men with an easy excuse to avoid changing their behavior.

Fact Or Fiction?

There is no way to predict who will be an abuser.

Fact: A number of factors serve as "red flags." According to Richard J. Gelles, an expert on domestic abuse, homes with two of the following factors have twice the violence of those where none of these factors are present. In homes with seven of the factors, violence is 40 times as likely. Those factors include:

- Previous involvement with domestic violence
- An unemployed husband
- A husband who uses illegal drugs at least once a year
- Spouses who are of different religions
- A husband who as a child witnessed his father hit his mother
- A husband who did not graduate from high school
- A husband who is between 18 and 30 years old
- A spouse who is violent toward children in the home
- Household income below the poverty level
- A husband employed at a job that involves unskilled labor
- A couple that live together but are not married

SOCIOLOGICAL THEORIES

Sociological theories look to larger forces, such as the attitudes of society as a whole, to explain the dynamics of abuse. Feminist theory, for example, sees abuse as a result of unequal power between men and women. This theory was first put forward in the 1979 book *Violence against Wives: A Case against the Patriarchy.* The book's authors, R. Emerson Dobash and Russell Dobash, argue that women have been subjugated by men throughout history, and their lack of power places them at the mercy of men. According to feminist theory, women's powerlessness extends to their relationships and that allows men to feel free to treat their wives as they please.

Resource theory and other theories inspired by it suggest that all family members use some degree of force to make sure other members meet their needs. According to resource theory, families are tied together through transactions or exchanges. The head of the household provides money, food, shelter, and clothing to the other members in return for respect, obedience, and maintenance of the household. According to this theory, people in lower social classes have fewer resources to exchange and therefore less power. Their powerlessness leads to frustration and bitterness that can erupt into violence. This theory suggests that poor people experience higher levels of abuse, a finding that has real-world support, especially when it comes to **child abuse**.

Social learning theory, developed by psychologist Albert Bandura, argues that children learn behavior such as abuse by imitating the actions of parents or **caregivers**. Children who observe their parents fighting or solving problems through the use of force are likely to grow up seeing those behaviors as acceptable ways of dealing with frustration. The *Journal of Family Violence* in 1990 reported a study that linked family violence by parents to later family violence by their children. A 1989 paper titled "Generalization and Containment: Different Effects of Past Aggression for Wives and Husbands" showed that family violence witnessed by a child may be transferred to other relationships over time.

Peers—friends or acquaintances of one's own age—can also be an important agent in socializing a child toward or away from violence. The article "Social Incompetence and the Intergenerational Transmission of Abusive Parental Practices" says that peer attitudes and actions can encourage or discourage a child from continuing to model violent behavior witnessed at home. Nevertheless, social learning theory still sees the family as the main socializing agent. That is, most people still learn basic standards of conduct and morality at home. Social learning theory also holds that these lessons are the most important in shaping an individual's social development.

Murray Straus's conflict theory suggests that conflict is actually needed to ensure the proper functioning of a family. He maintains that suppressing conflict causes a build-up of hostile feelings that can undermine the stability of the family. Avoiding conflict actually increases the likelihood of violent eruptions when peace can no longer be maintained.

According to the 1980 article "Culture, Social Organization and the Irony in the Study of Family Violence," conflict is more likely within the family than within other groups because a family's activities touch on all aspects of a person's life. Other groups operate within much more limited areas. Spouses, in particular, have a large number of interactions about a wide variety of matters, thus increasing the potential for conflict and violence.

According to conflict theory, outside factors such as stress, unemployment, or a previous history of family violence increase the likelihood of violent behavior. The nature of the power-sharing relationship between spouses also has an impact. A 1986 article titled "Marital Power, Conflict, and Violence in a Nationally Representative Sample of American Couples" found lower rates of conflict in couples where the wife and husband shared power and decision making more evenly and higher rates when one partner was dominant. Interestingly, the findings were the same regardless of which partner was dominant—husband or wife. The inequality of power sharing was more important than who held the power.

Stress theory claims that changes in family structure cause stress that leads to conflict. Such changes include marriage, the arrival of children, retirement, and aging. The 1986 article "The Application of Stress Theory to the Study of Family Violence" claims that American families are not well equipped to deal with the many stressors that they encounter. As more sources of stress accumulate, the family has a particularly difficult time coping in nonviolent ways.

Sociological theories of abuse have been criticized for providing an incomplete picture of the root causes of abuse. For example, they ignore the role of emotions such as anger and frustration in producing abuse. In addition, they assume that violence is learned and outline principles involved in that learning. However, those same principles could be applied to learning to control violence. However, no sociological theories have explored that aspect of social learning. Finally, much of the data to support such theories comes from the recollection of victims or abusers long after the abuse has occurred. Thus, the information on which the theories are based may be inaccurate or unreliable.

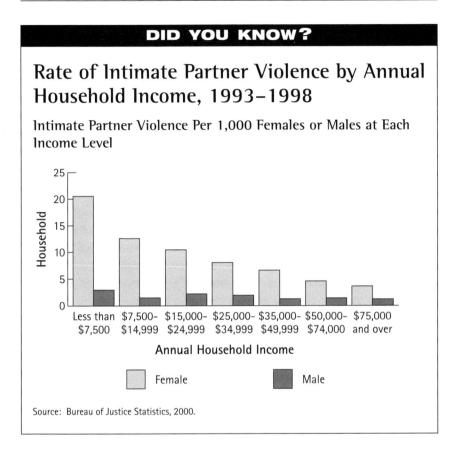

DID YOU KNOW?

Rate of Intimate Partner Violence by Annual Household Income, 1993–1998

Intimate Partner Violence Per 1,000 Females or Males at Each Income Level

Annual Household Income

Female   Male

Source: Bureau of Justice Statistics, 2000.

INTEGRATING THE THEORIES

A group called People Who Work With People Who Batter has tried to integrate ideas from many of the theories outlined. According to the organization, most abuse workers can agree that domestic violence exhibits the following traits:

- It is an issue for individuals, families, and the community. It is also a cultural and spiritual issue.
- It is learned behavior with rewards and consequences.
- It is reinforced by the media, legal system, and other institutions.
- It is based on the misuse of power and the desire to control another person.

■ It is a choice for which the abuser must be held accountable. Batterers can learn to make nonviolent choices.

Regardless of its root causes, abuse is a serious issue that requires families to work together to stop it. It is unlikely that a single theory can explain the various internal and external factors that may lead to abuse. However, these theories can provide clues for therapists and counselors in determining the most effective treatment and prevention strategies. For that reason, researchers are likely to continue to advance new theories to account for the many potential sources of abusive behavior.

See also: Abuse, Witnesses of; Abusers, Common Traits of; Domestic Partner Abuse; Men and Abuse; Women and Abuse

FURTHER READING

Bagley, Christopher, Kanka Mallick, and the Center for Evaluative and Developmental Research. *Child Sexual Abuse and Adult Offenders: New Theory and Research.* Williston, VT: Ashgate Publishing Company, 1999.

Bennett, Gary. *Elder Abuse: Concepts, Theories, and Interventions.* London: Chapman and Hall, 1994.

Harway, Michele. *What Causes Men's Violence against Women?* Thousand Oaks, CA: Sage Publications, 1999.

Mignon, Silvia I. *Family Abuse: Consequences, Theories, and Responses.* Boston: Allyn and Bacon, 2002.

■ ABUSE, WITNESSES OF

The effects of abuse are not limited to its victims. Children who witness abuse often suffer psychological trauma that can lead to a range of emotional and behavioral problems. There has long been speculation that witnesses and victims of abuse are more likely to become abusers themselves. While there is some evidence to suggest this may be the case, the issue is far from settled.

EFFECTS OF WITNESSING ABUSE

A number of research studies have examined the relationship between witnessing violence as a child and the development of behavioral, emotional, and cognitive problems. In "Problems Associated with Children's Witnessing of Domestic Violence," researcher Jeffrey Edelson reported that children who witnessed domestic violence scored higher on measures of antisocial and aggressive behaviors on certain questionnaires. The children also showed more fearful and inhibited behavior and were less socially competent than their **peers**.

Other problems experienced by children who witnessed domestic violence included greater levels of anxiety and **depression**, low self-esteem, and problems with temperament. Compared to children from nonviolent homes, they also tended to be less able to understand the feelings of others or to see things from another person's point of view. Male children who experienced serious violence at home had poorer peer relationships, less self-control, and less overall competence than children from nonabusive families.

Researchers have also found some evidence that witnessing abuse can result in cognitive and learning difficulties. A study published in the 1999 book *Children Exposed to Marital Violence* found that increased exposure to domestic violence may impair cognitive abilities such as reasoning, judgment, and problem solving. However a 1995 study titled "The Psychological Functioning of Children from Backgrounds of Domestic Violence" found no significant differences in academic abilities between children who witness abuse and those who do not.

Longer-term effects of witnessing abuse have been exhibited by adult victims many years after the abuse, as shown in a 1995 article published in the *Journal of Family Violence*. The study, which examined 550 undergraduate college students, found that those who had witnessed violence as children were more likely to suffer from depression, trauma, and low self-esteem.

Fact Or Fiction?

Children of different ages react differently to witnessing abuse.

Fact: According to Karen Nielsen at The Family Centre in Edmonton, Alberta, preschoolers who witness abuse are likely to yell, be irritable, stutter, and have nightmares or other sleep disturbances. Those under age 10 also often blame themselves for the violence. Adolescents display more aggressive behavior, abuse drugs or alcohol, or attempt suicide. They don't typically blame themselves for the violence, but they often excuse the abuser's behavior. An older child may even be angry with the abused spouse for putting up with the punishment. However, there are some similarities in the reactions of children exposed to abuse, regardless of age. Both may act out the role of either the abuser or the victim. Young boys may become bullies, and older boys may become abusive in dating relationships. Adolescent girls who witness abuse may enter abusive dating relationships.

FACTORS ASSOCIATED WITH WITNESSING VIOLENCE

Witnessing domestic violence does not have the same impact on all children. Characteristics of the child, as well as the relationship between the parents and child, can play a part in determining how the child is affected.

The child's age and sex seem to affect how a child reacts to seeing abuse. According to a 1988 article in the *American Journal of Orthopsychiatry*, preschool children who witness abuse report greater problems than older children. Boys and girls also tend to differ in their behavioral response to witnessing violence. The article cites studies that suggest boys who witness abuse generally show more external aggression and hostility, while girls more often show inward distress such as depression and physical complaints.

An article in the *Journal of Clinical and Consulting Psychology* titled "Children of Battered Women: The Relation of Child Behavior to Family Violence and Maternal Stress," suggested that a child's relationship with his or her mother is a key factor in determining how the child will respond to seeing domestic violence. The authors found that the higher the mother's level of stress, the greater the problems experienced by the children. Other studies, however, have called this finding into question. Nevertheless, family influences are seen as important factors in a child's reaction to viewing abuse. Edelson cites a 1994 study from the *American Journal of Public Health* that found black adolescents from stable households were less likely to suffer adverse effects from witnessing domestic violence compared with those from less stable homes.

DO THE ABUSED BECOME ABUSERS?

One very controversial and widely debated topic is whether children who are abused or witness abuse are more likely to become abusers themselves as adults. Those who support the idea of a connection between witnessing and enacting violence see abuse as a learned behavior. They argue that children model the violence they see at home and use the same behaviors when raising their own children. Opponents of the theory claim that there is no simple and direct relationship between witnessing or suffering abuse and becoming abusive.

As mentioned earlier, some children (particularly males) who witness domestic violence do exhibit higher levels of aggressive behavior in the short term. A 1996 study titled "Trends in a National Sample of Sexually Abusive Youth" suggested that those who suffer childhood sexual abuse are at greater risk of committing sexual crimes later in life. Of 1,600 youths in the study who had committed sexual offenses, 39.1 percent had been sexually abused as children, and 63.4 percent had witnessed violence at home.

However, this and other studies drawing similar conclusions have been criticized on a number of points. First, they rely on adult subjects to provide information based on events that they say occurred in the past. There is no way to verify the accuracy of these claims of past abuse or to know if the victims are accurately recalling the circumstances of the alleged abuse. Also, these studies do not examine other factors that might have played a role in the development of a person's later abusive behavior.

Q & A

Question: I've heard that children who are abused will grow up to be child abusers. Is that right?

Answer: This doesn't mean people who have been abused as children are programmed to become abusers. They can have healthy relationships and raise children. But because they experienced the physical and emotional strain of being abused, they may be very determined not to repeat the cycle. They may need counseling to avoid repeating the pattern established by their parents.

More recent studies have called into question the link between witnessing or experiencing abuse and becoming an abuser. In 1996, the General Accounting Office (GAO) issued a report to the U.S. Congress titled "Cycle of Sexual Abuse: Research Inconclusive about Whether Child Victims Become Adult Abusers." The report examined

25 studies into the question of whether abused children become adult abusers. Only two of those studies actually observed victims from the time they suffered abuse as children to adulthood. The remaining studies interviewed known adult sex offenders about past abuses. Studies of both types found that most offenders were not victims of childhood abuse.

These conclusions were supported by a 2003 report from the Institute of Child Health in London. That study found that few men who were sexually abused as children became child sex abusers themselves as adults. In the study, conducted by researcher David Skuse and his colleagues, only 26 of 224 former victims of **child sexual abuse** went on to commit sex crimes. The researchers in the study found that poor parental supervision, abuse by a female, and violence in the family did, however, increase the likelihood that the victim would later sexually abuse others.

The mixed results from these studies indicate the need for more research into the relationship between suffering and witnessing abuse and later committing abuse. Even those studies that show no direct link between the two suggest that there may be more complex connections that lead from victim to perpetrator. Researchers are still seeking a more thorough understanding of whether and how abuse is passed from one generation to another.

See also: Abuse, Theories of; Abusers, Common Traits of; Child Abuse; Child Sexual Abuse; Domestic Partner Abuse; Post-traumatic Stress Disorder and Abuse

■ ABUSERS, COMMON TRAITS OF

Abusers are people who use physical, verbal, or emotional violence to control the behavior of others. Perhaps the two most common forms of abuse are domestic partner abuse and child abuse. People who abuse their domestic partners (a person, not necessarily a spouse, with whom one cohabits and shares a long-term sexual relationship) or children are hard to spot. To most outsiders, they seem "regular," "normal," even very likeable and charming. In public these individuals may seem loving and attentive to their partners or children. The abuse occurs in private and close family members may try to hide it.

Other members of the family may be shocked when they find out a relative is abusive to a partner or child.

Given that it is impossible to identify an abuser from outward appearances, it is important to recognize signs that suggest a person may be prone to abusive behavior. Some of these signs are internal traits such as attitudes or ways of handling emotions. Others are external indicators, such as violent behavior or a family history of abuse. Knowing what to look for can help you avoid becoming involved in an abusive relationship.

CHARACTERISTICS OF
DOMESTIC PARTNER ABUSERS

Abusers can be found in every economic group, race, and ethnic group. They include those who live in million-dollar homes and people who have barely a nickel to their names. Despite their diversity, many abusers share certain psychological traits. Various national agencies have identified a group of warning signs that indicate those who are more likely to become abusers:

- A history of witnessing or experiencing domestic abuse. Many abusers were possibly victims of childhood abuse or witnesses to domestic violence. According to a 1993 article in the *American Journal of Orthopsychiatry*, a high proportion of violent men—and their victims—were raised in violent homes and witnessed domestic abuse as children. In 1984 the *Journal of Marriage and the Family* reported similar findings. In fact, that study found that children who witnessed violence between their parents were even more likely to become domestic abusers than children who were actually abused.

- Low self-esteem. The National Council on Child Abuse and Family Violence (NCCAFV) and the National Coalition Against Domestic Violence (NCADV) both report that **batterers** generally have low self-esteem. While they may seem outwardly successful and confident, abusers often feel they are failures. They may express their frustration and anger about failure through violent behavior.

- Uncontrolled temper. An abusive person is unable to tolerate frustration and has what experts call "poor impulse control." The *1999 National Victim Assistance Academy* reports that many abusers have not learned how to express feelings such as anger, frustration, or guilt in a healthy fashion. Instead, they express these emotions through violence. This violent temper may not be apparent to friends or coworkers because abusers usually do a good job of keeping it bottled up in public. The abuse, whether physical, emotional, or verbal, typically happens at home, out of sight.

■ Possessiveness and controlling behavior. According to the NCADV, domestic abusers tend to treat women as objects or possessions. They feel a sense of ownership over their partners and try to control their activities and behaviors. For example, abusers may not let their partners make any financial or personal decisions, or they may control the family money and use of the car. Abusers may eventually isolate their partners by cutting off ties to family and friends.

■ Intense fear of abandonment. Because of their low self-esteem, abusers often live in fear that their partners will abandon them. That fear can lead to behavior intended to control the partner so that he or she cannot leave.

■ Extreme jealousy. The National Center for Post-Traumatic Stress Disorder (NCPTSD) and the NCADV report that abusers are often jealous of time their partners spend with other people. This usually stems from their fear of abandonment and need to control their partner's behavior.

■ Inability to accept responsibility for their own behavior. According to the NCADV, abusers often blame some outside factor for their abuse. For example, abusers may claim that a stressful day or drinking set off the abuse. Abusers also often blame their victims, claiming that the victim did or said something that triggered the abuse. The abusers refuse to see that the real problem is their own inappropriate reaction to their partners. In other cases, abusers may deny that the abuse occurred or minimize its seriousness.

Fact Or Fiction?

Only straight women are battered.

Fact: Although the majority of domestic abuse involves a man battering a female partner, about five percent of the battering in heterosexual relationships is committed by the woman toward her male partner. In addition, a man can also be battered by his gay partner, and a woman by her lesbian partner. Research on same-sex domestic violence can be difficult given the fact that many gays and lesbians are not open about their relationships, including abusive ones. Research reported by the National Coalition of Anti-Violence Programs (NCAVP) indicates that battering in same-sex relationships is about as common as in heterosexual relationships. In its report *Lesbian, Gay, Bisexual, and Transgender Domestic Violence, 2001,* the NCAVP reports that abuse occurs in 15–20 percent of all gay relationships. In 2001 there were 5,046 reported incidents of domestic violence among lesbian, gay, and bisexual individuals, an increase of some 25 percent over the previous year. One of the studies summarized in the report called domestic abuse "the third most severe health problem facing gay men today."

The NCPTSD identifies three other warning signs of a potential abuser:

- Quick involvement. Abusers may come on very strong at first and pressure their partners to move quickly into intimate relationships.
- Cruelty to animals and children. Abusers often are insensitive to the pain and suffering of children and animals. They may tease animals or children cruelly or expect children to be able to do things beyond their age, ability, or understanding.
- Wide mood swings. Abusers may feel great remorse for their actions and promise to change if their partner doesn't leave. Abusers may even become particularly kind and loving for a time. However, this "honeymoon" period in a pattern of abuse is short-lived. The tension builds, violence erupts once again, and the attacks can become more severe over time.

Q & A

Question: What are the warning signs that a person may become a batterer?

Answer: According to the National Coalition Against Domestic Violence, there are several signs that may predict whether a man (or woman) will be a batterer:

- Did he (or she) grow up in a violent family?
- Does he use violence to solve problems?
- Does he have a substance abuse problem?
- Does he have strong beliefs in stereotypical roles for men and women?
- Is he jealous of his partner's other interests and relationships?
- Does he have access to weapons?
- Does he expect his partner to follow his orders?
- Does he have severe mood swings?
- Does he cause his partner to fear him?
- Does he treat his partner roughly?

DRUG AND ALCOHOL ABUSE

Research shows a relationship between alcohol abuse and domestic violence. A study published in the *Alcohol Treatment Quarterly* in 1984 showed that over half of the **battered** wives calling a Philadelphia-area hotline said their husbands had been drinking at the time of the abuse. However, researchers have yet to prove a direct relationship between alcohol abuse and violent behavior. Despite the lack of a direct connection, many men blame drugs and alcohol for their abusive behavior. In many cases, this is a way to avoid taking responsibility for their own violence.

Other studies have shown that a pattern of family alcohol or drug use puts a person at greater risk of becoming an abuser. According to a 1988 study "Personality and Biographical Data That Characterize Men Who Abuse Their Wives," children exposed to alcoholism, drug abuse, and family violence were more likely to abuse their spouses as adults. The *Journal of Mental and Nervous Disease* reported a 1983 study that

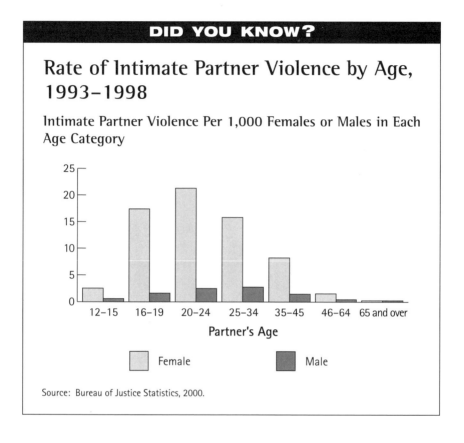

DID YOU KNOW?

Rate of Intimate Partner Violence by Age, 1993–1998

Intimate Partner Violence Per 1,000 Females or Males in Each Age Category

Partner's Age

Female   Male

Source: Bureau of Justice Statistics, 2000.

also found a connection between exposure to family alcohol and drug abuse and the risk of later spouse abuse. According to the study, men who were raised in a family where one or more parents abused alcohol or drugs were more likely to abuse their spouses as adults.

CHARACTERISTICS OF CHILD ABUSERS

By definition, the people who commit child abuse or **neglect** are the very people responsible for the child's safety and well-being: parents, other relatives, guardians, baby-sitters, or other caretakers. Neglect occurs when a caretaker does not provide adequate food, shelter, medical care, or supervision. Neglect also involves a parent or guardian failing to take care of a child's emotional needs, exposing a child to danger such as domestic violence, or leaving a very young child alone in the house.

A parent's age, income, and marital status are important factors in child abuse or neglect. According to the World Health Organization's

(WHO) 2002 *World Report on Violence and Health*, parents who are young, poor, unemployed, and/or single are more likely to abuse their children. WHO reports that single mothers commit more child abuse in the United States than any other group. The person most likely to batter a child is the child's own mother.

According to the Department of Health and Human Services, mothers perpetrated 40.3 percent of all child abuse violations in 2002. The mother and father together were responsible for a further 18 percent of all child abuse, and the mother together with someone other than the father committed about 5 percent of child abuse violations. In total, mothers were involved in nearly two out of every three cases of child abuse reported in the United States in 2002.

Child abuse often stems from the financial and emotional stresses of raising children. Abusers may love their children but feel isolated and lack needed financial and emotional support. Neglect and abuse may also occur when parents do not understand a child's needs and abilities at various stages in his or her development. Parent may not understand why their baby won't stop crying, why a toddler can't just sit still, or why five-year-olds can't make their own lunches.

People who were abused or who witnessed family violence as children are more likely to commit child abuse as adults. Child abuse is also more likely in homes where partner abuse is also occurring. Some of the same traits that lead husbands or boyfriends to batter their partners, such as an inability to control their temper or a need to control others around them, may also result in their battering a child. Tragically, this pattern is often repeated in the next generation. Research shows that parents who grew up in violent households are more likely to commit violence against their own children.

TEENS SPEAK

My Name Is Eric, and I Have a Serious Issue at Home

I don't talk about it much at school or to my friends, because I'm embarrassed and I don't want a lot of people knowing about it. The problem is with my folks. My dad is really mean to my mom sometimes, and they get into some terrible arguments. It usually starts over something small, like a disagreement over housework or some errand my dad forgot to run. All of a sudden, he's yelling and screaming at my mom, calling her all sorts of names. Sometimes he gets violent, knocking things over, throwing stuff around the house, and even hitting my mom or me.

It's really scary, and sometimes I worry that he's going to hurt my mom or me. Then, a little while later, I'll hear him apologize to my mom and tell her it will never happen again. Sometimes I hear him crying and even begging her to forgive him. I think he's scared she might leave. I'm scared about that too. My dad's behavior is frightening sometimes, but the idea of splitting up the family is just as scary. What would we do without my dad? My mom doesn't work, and I can't take care of us by myself.

I talked to my counselor at school, and she said that I need to try to get my dad and mom to talk to a counselor about their problems. She also said it was good that I came to see her, because I need someone to talk to as well. She warned me that kids who grow up in a violent family can become violent to their own families later on in life. She said that I need to be aware of my feelings so I can learn how to deal with my own anger and frustration in positive ways. I'm going to keep talking to my counselor. I want to help my dad stop hurting my mom and me, and I sure don't want to hurt my family when I become an adult.

The first step to avoiding a destructive pattern of behavior such as child or partner abuse is recognizing the warning signs. If you notice any of the characteristics of abusers in yourself, seek advice on how to deal with those behaviors and attitudes before they grow into a pattern of abuse. If you know someone who exhibits the warning signs of abusive behavior, talk to him or her about the behavior or ask friends and family to help you talk with the individual. The best solution to domestic abuse and child abuse is to address such issues early and prevent the problem before it starts.

See also: Abuse, Theories of; Abuse, Witnesses of; Child Abuse, Domestic Partner Abuse; Men and Abuse; Women and Abuse

FURTHER READING
Dutton, Donald G. *The Abusive Personality: Violence and Control in Intimate Relationships.* New York: Guilford Publications, 2002.
Dutton, Donald G., and Susan K. Golant. *The Batterer: A Psychological Profile.* New York: Basic Books, 1997.

■ ALCOHOL, DRUGS, AND ABUSE

The nonmedical use of a substance in order to affect one's mental processes, to satisfy a dependence (an intense physical or psychological need for a substance), or to attempt suicide. Alcohol and drug abuse are serious problems in the United States not only because of their direct effects on the health of the user but also because they contribute to other societal problems. Alcohol and drugs play a significant role in initiating and facilitating abusive behavior. The abuse of alcohol and other drugs has been linked to aggression, crime, and many types of abusive behavior. Abusing alcohol or drugs can also increase one's chances of being a victim of abuse as well as a perpetrator or abuser.

ALCOHOL AND DRUG EFFECTS

To understand how alcohol and drugs can contribute to aggression and abuse, it is necessary to understand how these substances affect the body and brain. Alcohol is a central nervous system **depressant**, which means it slows down certain bodily functions controlled by the nervous system. These functions include breathing, reaction time, and decision-making skills. Alcohol also lowers inhibitions, which increases the likelihood of taking risks that one would avoid when sober. A person under the influence of alcohol thus has a reduced capacity to make reasoned judgments. He or she is more likely to make a rash decision. Other common depressants include drugs such as **barbiturates**, PCP (phencyclidine), and methaquaalone (Quaaludes).

Although a large number of violent crimes are committed under the influence of alcohol, alcohol does not *cause* violent behavior. Instead researchers suggest that by clouding judgment and reducing inhibitions, alcohol seems to increase the chances that one will act in an aggressive or violent manner. A classic 1975 study titled "Effects of Alcohol on Aggression in Male Social Drinkers" found that expectations play a significant role in the link between alcohol and aggression. Subjects in the study were given a nonalcoholic drink, but some were told it was alcohol and others were told that it was not. Subjects who believed the drink was alcoholic acted more aggressively than those who knew it was nonalcoholic.

Depressants are not the only types of drugs associated with aggressive behavior. **Stimulants** such as **cocaine, amphetamines,** and **methamphetamines** have also been linked to violence. These substances increase the activity of the central nervous system, which can produce feelings of irritability, apprehensiveness, and **paranoia** (extreme and unreasonable feelings of persecution). Users may reach an extremely agitated state in which they are more likely to react violently to situations they perceive as annoying or threatening.

Fact Or Fiction?

People can't help what they do under the influence of alcohol.

Fact: Alcohol impairs judgment, motor skills, and other behavior, but Canadian researchers have found that drinkers can sober up quickly with the right motivation. In a 2001 study conducted by the University of Waterloo in Ontario, researchers asked volunteers to press a button when prompted by the computer screen. The subjects were told not to respond if a red light also appeared. The people under the influence of alcohol were more likely to press the button, even if the red light appeared. However, when the drinkers were offered a small reward for their performance, they behaved as well as the sober subjects. This study indicates that, if properly motivated, people can exercise control over their behavior while under the influence of alcohol.

SUBSTANCE USE AND VIOLENCE

Although substance use may not directly cause violence, studies have shown a strong connection between the two. According to *Violence and Drug Abuse,* a 1995 publication by the National Institute on Drug Abuse, alcohol abuse is a factor in approximately 50 percent of the violent crimes committed in the United States, including about 15 percent of all homicides (murders). Cocaine, amphetamines, and methamphetamines are also drugs that have been linked to aggressive behavior and hostility, but statistics from the Federal Bureau of

Investigation's *Uniform Crime Reports* shows that less than 5 percent of all homicides are related to drugs other than alcohol.

Substance abuse has also been associated with violence among teens. In 2001, the Department of Health and Human Services (HHS) reported that teens who participated in violent activities during the previous year were more likely to use alcohol and illicit drugs than nonviolent teens. The HHS report found that 85 percent of violent teens used **marijuana,** and 55 percent used several illegal drugs. Teen drug users reported higher rates for a range of violent behaviors such as gang fights, fighting at school or work, and attacking others with the intent of seriously harming them. In 2003 the Web site www.teen-violence.com reported that 25 percent of all teen violence occurs under the influence of drugs or alcohol.

Q & A

Question: After having a few drinks at a party I got into an argument with a friend that almost ended up in a fight. I never act like that when I'm sober. Was it the alcohol that made me lose my temper?

Answer: Although studies have linked alcohol and aggression, there is no proof that drinking causes violent behavior. However, drinking does break down inhibitions and impair judgment. This may make you more likely to express your feelings in inappropriate or unfamiliar ways. If you are concerned about the way you behave under the influence of alcohol, your drinking could be a problem. Talk to an adult about your drinking—as well as your aggressive behavior—and seek help for both.

SUBSTANCE USE AND ABUSIVE BEHAVIOR

According to a 1998 study sponsored by the National Center of Addiction and Substance Abuse at Columbia University, parental substance abuse has produced "chaos, collapse, and calamity, leaving behind a wreckage of millions of children." In the study, which interviewed 915 child-welfare professionals, 80 percent of those who responded said substance abuse either causes or plays a role in most cases of child abuse (the use of physical or emotional violence to control the behavior of a child). Forty percent of those interviewed said that substance abuse contributed to more than three-quarters of the child abuse cases they handle. In addition, 70 percent of the professionals said that substance abuse was one of the three leading factors responsible for the doubling of the rate of child abuse in the United States between 1986 and 1997.

Other research suggests that alcohol is the drug most commonly associated with domestic partner abuse (the use of physical or emotional violence to control a domestic partner). This connection was examined in a 1984 article in the journal *Alcohol Treatment Quarterly* titled "Alcohol-Related Domestic Violence: Clinical Implications and Intervention Strategies." The article reported the results of a study of 1,500 cases of abused wives who had called a help hotline in Philadelphia. More than half of the women interviewed (55 percent) said their husbands became abusive toward them after drinking. This finding is of particular concern for families with children, because research has shown that children of abusive parents are at greater risk of becoming child and spouse abusers themselves. According to the 1983 article "Men Who Batter: Some Personality Characteristics," boys who are raised by one or more abusive parents are more likely to abuse their spouses as adults.

The National Committee for the Prevention of Elder Abuse (NCPEA) reports that drug and alcohol abuse is the risk factor most often cited for elder abuse (the mistreatment of a dependent elderly person). According to the NCPEA, substance abusers may see elderly relatives as a source of money for their drug habit or may use their homes as a base for drug dealing. In addition, the NCPEA found that elderly spouses who abuse their partners are more likely to be violent under the influence of alcohol or drugs.

Substance abuse—particularly drinking—is a part of many instances of hazing (playing humiliating pranks on an individual as a form of initiation into a club or other group). According to Alfred University's 1999 study "Initiation Rites in American High Schools: A National Survey," 23 percent of U.S. high school students who were subjected to hazing were asked to participate in substance abuse. Of the students surveyed, 24 percent of boys and 18 percent of girls reported that substance abuse was part of the hazing ritual.

Alcohol and drug use also play a key role in dating abuse. In 1993 the *Journal of Sex Education and Therapy* reported the results of a study that found 67.5 percent of college males who sexually assaulted their dates had been drinking. Drug and alcohol use increases the chances of suffering dating abuse as well as committing it. Research cited by the National Center for Injury Prevention and Control shows that both the frequency and seriousness of injuries increase with greater intake of alcohol or drugs by either the abuser or the victim.

A particular subject of concern relating to dating and substance abuse is the issue of **date rape drugs**. The three most common date rape drugs are Rohypnol, GHB (gamma hydroxybutyrate), and keta-mine. When slipped into a drink, a date rape drug renders one uncon-scious and helpless to defend oneself against date rape. In addition, the victim of a date rape drug typically has no recollection of what happened. These drugs are odorless and tasteless, which makes them very difficult for the victim to detect in a drink.

Date rape drugs generally fall in the category of **depressants** because of their effects on the central nervous system. These drugs are particularly dangerous when combined with alcohol, another depres-sant. Together, the two drugs may depress breathing and heart rate to such dangerously low levels that they may result in respiratory fail-ure, coma, and death.

SUBSTANCE USE AND VICTIMIZATION

Alcohol and drugs not only increase one's chances of committing vio-lence or abuse, they also increase one's chances of being a victim. According to the 1992 article "Post-traumatic Stress Disorder among Substance Users from the General Population," marijuana users were 46 percent more likely to be assaulted than people who did not use drugs. Users of harder drugs such as **heroin**, cocaine, and ampheta-mines were 40 percent more likely to suffer assault.

The 1997 National Institute of Justice research preview *Drugs, Alcohol, and Domestic Violence in Memphis* reported that 42 percent of domestic violence victims had used alcohol or drugs on the day they were assaulted. Some 15 percent of those victims had used cocaine, and about half of those who had used it were forced to do so by their attacker. According to a 1994 study by the United States Department of Justice titled "Murder in Families, Special Report," half of the homicide victims murdered by their spouses used alcohol before the crime.

In 1998 the Bureau of Justice Statistics reported that drinking by the perpetrator or the victim occurs in over half of all rapes and sex-ual assaults. A study published the previous year in the *Journal of Consulting and Clinical Psychology* found that drug use increased a woman's chances of being sexually assaulted. According to "A Two-Year Longitudinal Analysis of the Relationships between Violent Assault and Substance Use in Women," use of drugs nearly doubled the likelihood that a woman would experience an assault when compared with those who did not use drugs. Those at greatest risk were women who used drugs and had experienced a previous assault.

Substance abuse can even undermine the victim's attempts to get help. The 1988 book *Violence in America: A Public Health Approach* found that victims of domestic partner abuse who use drugs and alcohol may not be taken as seriously by police or other law enforcement officials. According to another 1988 publication, *Health Education and Feminist Strategy: The Case of Woman Abuse,* officials may view the victim's substance abuse as the reason he or she was abused.

In addition to increasing one's chances of victimization, substance abuse can be a signal that a person is suffering from abuse. According to *Violence in America,* women who have been physically or sexually assaulted are twice as likely to use or abuse drugs and alcohol as those who were not assaulted. "Assault, Abuse, and Axis I Comorbidity," a 1992 study published by the American Psychiatric Association, reported that 65 percent of female substance abusers surveyed had been sexually assaulted. In the 1999 National Treatment Improvement Evaluation Study, 43 percent of the adult women receiving substance abuse treatment reported having been sexually abused.

Even though the links between substance abuse, aggression, and abuse are indirect, they are significant enough to be a source of concern. Any outside factor such as substance abuse that can increase the risk of becoming a perpetrator or victim of abuse should be avoided. It is much easier to make the right decisions about relationships, dating, sexual behavior, and caring for **dependents** without the influence of drugs or alcohol.

See also: Abusers, Common Traits of; Child Abuse; Dating Abuse; Domestic Partner Abuse; Elder Abuse; Hazing; Sexual Abuse; Sexual Assault

FURTHER READING
Hampton, Robert L., Vincent Senatore, and Thomas Gulotta. *Substance Abuse, Family Violence, and Child Welfare: Bridging Perspectives.* Thousand Oaks, CA: Sage Publications, 1998.

Jamiolkowski, Raymond M. *Drugs and Domestic Violence*. New York: Rosen Publishing Group, 1995.

Wekerle, Christine, and Anne Marie Wall. *The Violence and Addiction Equation: Theoretical and Clinical Issues in Substance Abuse and Relationship Violence*. New York: Brunner-Routledge, 2001.

■ BULLYING

Bullying involves repeated and systematic attacks by a more powerful person or group on a less powerful one. Bullying includes a wide range of actions, including physical violence, name-calling and insults, teasing, humiliation, verbal or written threats, and extortion (intimidating someone to get money or other valuables from them). To be considered a bully, these behaviors must occur more than once and must be intended to frighten the victim.

TEENS SPEAK

I Was Only 12 Years Old When Something Ugly Happened to Me

I thought that by the time I was in seventh grade I would be one of the "big kids," someone who got to walk around like they owned the school. Instead, I snuck around school trying to fly under the radar.

The harassment began with whispers whenever I walked by these four boys. They began making ugly antigay comments. Then the harassment got physical. They began to trip me when I went by, and they pushed me into the lockers and yelled comments at me. Other kids stood around when that happened, as if they didn't know what to do. There weren't any teachers around, but I had never seen them stop anyone from making antigay comments.

It just kept getting worse. One time they jumped me in the bathroom and pushed my head in a urinal. Another time, they came up behind me after school and put a rope noose around my neck and pulled it tight. I thought I was going to die then, but after about 35 seconds, I managed to loosen the noose.

It didn't end until they threatened to bring a gun to school and shoot me and my best friend. They thought he was my boyfriend. A student overheard this and told a teacher. The teacher reported it to the principal, and she called the police.

I don't know why people are so uptight about gays and lesbians. I don't understand why the teachers don't stop the hate language the instant they hear it. They hit the roof if they hear racial or religious slurs, but gay harassment is still okay!

INCIDENCE OF BULLYING

Research conducted since the 1980s has revealed that bullying is a widespread problem. Dan Olweus, perhaps the world's leading authority on bullying, conducted some of the first extensive studies in Norway. After conducting research for more than 20 years, he has found that about 15 percent of students experience problems with bullying. About 9 percent are victims of bullying, while the remainder bully others regularly. About 3 percent of the students Olweus studied were victimized at least once a week. Two percent of students bullied others at least once a week.

Research has revealed even higher levels of bullying in the United States. In 1995, the National Education Association (NEA) estimated that 160,000 students miss school every day because they fear being bullied by another student. That same year, the National Center for Education Statistics reported that 77 percent of middle school and high school students in small Midwestern towns had been bullied. According to a 2001 study from the National Institute of Child Health and Human Development (NICHD), almost one-third of students in grades six through 10 bully or are bullied. This represents a total 5.7 million children in the United States.

The NICHD study found that 29 percent of all students surveyed were involved in bullying, either as perpetrators or victims. According to the study, 10.6 percent of the children surveyed had "sometimes" bullied, others, while 8.8 percent bullied others at least once per week. About one in 12 students (8.5 percent) said they were "sometimes" bullied, and 8.4 percent were bullied at least once a week. Interestingly, 6.3 percent of students reported that they both bullied others and were themselves targets of bullying. Bullying occurred most often in sixth through eighth grades, and there was little difference in rates of bullying between urban, suburban, and rural schools.

Studies from several countries reveal that boys are more likely to be both the perpetrators and the victims of bullying. In his 1999 book *Bullying at School: What We Know and What We Can Do*, Olweus reports that 80 percent of boys and 60 percent of girls who were victims of bullying in grades five through seven were bullied only by boys. About 15–20 percent of girls were bullied by both girls and boys.

Olweus also found that verbal abuse is the most commonly used form of bullying by both boys and girls. Boys are more likely than girls to use physical violence, while girls more often use indirect bullying, such as shunning or gossiping about the victim. However, according to the 1994 article "Sex Differences in Physical, Verbal, and Indirect Aggression: A Review of Recent Research," boys use indirect bullying more often as their verbal skills increase.

DID YOU KNOW?

School Bullying Among Teens

Percentage of Students Ages 12–18 Who Reported Being Bullied at School During the Previous Six Months, by Grade Level and Gender: 1999

Note: "At school" means in the school building, on the school grounds, or on a school bus

Source: U.S. Department of Justice, 1999.

CHARACTERISTICS OF BULLIES AND VICTIMS

As with most forms of abuse, there is no simple answer to the question "What causes bullying?" However, researchers have identified several factors related to individual personality and the family environment that may increase the chances that a person will become a bully or victim.

According to Olweus and other researchers, certain childrearing styles may increase or decrease the chances of one becoming a bully. Children who experience little attention or warmth from parents, those whose parents engage in aggressive behavior at home, and those who do not have proper adult supervision are at greater risk of becoming bullies. Children who are active and impulsive by nature, and those who are physically stronger than their **peers** may also be more likely to bully others, even though most physically powerful children do not bully.

Victims of bullying tend to fall into two broad categories whose members exhibit some common traits. The Parent-Teacher Association of America (PTA) and ASAP (A School-based Anti-violence Program) call these categories "passive" victims and "reactive" victims. Passive bullying victims tend to be quiet, shy, and not confident in their physical strength. They often lack close friends or systems of social support at school. When bullied, the passive victim cries or runs away instead of fighting back.

By contrast, the reactive victim actually provokes attacks by being disruptive, irritating, or argumentative with other students. When bullied, the reactive victim fights back instead of withdrawing. Reactive victims sometimes bully other children, thus becoming both victim and bully. Olweus found that reactive victims, like bullies, tend to be impulsive. However, like passive victims, they typically have poor social skills.

Fact Or Fiction?

If people just stood up to bullies, the bullying would end.

Fact: Bullies victimize people who are weaker and less confident of their ability to defend themselves, so victims alone typically cannot stop the physical, emotional, or social violence. In addition, even reactive victims who fight back continue to be bullied. In order to end bullying, victims need adults and peers as allies. School officials and teachers need to take a stand against bullying, and schools must implement policies that punish bullies and teach them how to stop bullying.

THE EFFECTS OF BULLYING

According to ASAP, bullying victims typically experience fear, anxiety, and low self-esteem. Victims may also suffer psychological harm that negatively impacts their social, emotional, and academic development. The PTA found that bullying victims suffer more health problems and score lower in tests measuring academic achievement and self-esteem. As the 1995 National Education Association (NEA) study showed, fear of bullying causes many students to avoid school. Bullying also has long-term consequences. Olweus found that, as adults, male victims of bullying continued to experience lower self-esteem and were more likely to suffer from **depression** than those who were not bullied. Olweus reported on several cases of boys in Norway who had committed suicide as a result of bullying.

Bullies, too, suffer negative consequences from their actions. According to the NICHD study, bullies fared poorly in school and experienced other problem behaviors such as smoking cigarettes and drinking alcohol. The PTA reported that bullies often fail to develop coping skills and the ability to control their emotions, which can lead to difficulty adjusting to the demands of adult life. Bullies may also experience problems when establishing close relationships that are not based on fear or aggression. As adults they may be at a greater risk of abusing their spouses or children. Olweus found that bullies tend to grow into aggressive adults who are more likely to commit multiple criminal acts.

A third group that is affected by bullying are those who witness bullying. According to *School Safety Facts*, a 2003 publication by the NEA, bullying leads to a climate of fear and disrespect for authority in schools. Bullying impacts overall student behavior and learning. In addition, ASAP reports that many bystanders who would not bully on their own may follow a bully's lead in harassing another student. Children who witness aggressive bullying may be more likely to use aggression in the future, especially if they see no punishment or negative consequences associated with bullying.

RESPONDING TO BULLYING

Although bullying is clearly a serious problem, it is one that often goes unrecognized. In their 1997 book *Understanding Bullying at School: What Can We Do about It?*, authors Wendy Craig and Debra Pepler found that adults are often not aware that bullying is taking place in their children's schools. Even when parents and teachers are aware of bullying, many do not take it seriously or do nothing to prevent it. According to a 2002 article by the National Mental Health and Education Center titled "What Schools and Parents Can Do," 25 percent of teachers do not consider bullying, insults, or verbal harassment to be problem behaviors. As a result, only 4 percent of the teachers surveyed for the article intervened in cases of bullying. Many students are aware that adults are often ignorant about or apathetic toward bullying. The 2003 study *Findings from the Massachusetts Bullying Prevention Initiative* reported that 30 percent of the students in 14 Massachusetts schools felt that adults did little or nothing to stop bullying.

One of the first steps in responding to bullying is identifying when a child is being bullied. The PTA lists the following signs that parents and other adults should look for:

- Changes in the child's behavior, such as becoming more withdrawn or anxious
- Loss of interest in school or favorite activities
- Bruises, scratches, torn or dirty clothing, missing money, missing or damaged books or property
- Loss of appetite
- Frequent trips to the school nurse
- Sleeplessness, nightmares, crying in sleep
- Fear of going to school
- Frequent headaches or stomachaches, especially before school
- Taking roundabout or unfamiliar routes to school
- Reluctance to take the school bus
- Refusal to talk about the school day

If parents or adults believe that a child is being bullied, they should ask the child directly. ASAP also recommends that parents of bullied children try to get their children involved in social groups that provide positive social interactions. Belonging to such groups can be especially helpful if the victim is shy and has difficulty making friends. Such group activities can help him or her build competence, confidence, and self-esteem.

Schools should not only develop policies that deal with bullying but also react quickly when bullying occurs. ASAP recommends that school officials talk separately to the bully and victim. They should reassure the victim that they will prevent future bullying. They should not only punish the bully but also work to educate him or her about reducing aggressive behavior and becoming more aware of the feelings of others. Parents of both the bully and the victim should be notified as soon as possible. Parents should be involved in developing a plan to prevent future occurrences of bullying.

Q & A

Question: We learn in kindergarten not to be a "tattletale" or "snitch." Isn't that what I'd be if I reported bullying?

Answer: Reporting bullying is not "tattling" or "snitching." Bullying is a serious problem that can threaten someone's safety and should never be ignored. If you see someone being bullied, ask yourself these questions:

- Is there an immediate threat to anyone's safety?
- What is the responsible thing to do?
- Can the situation be resolved through direct communication with the person?
- If the bully is picking on someone other than you, have you tried to be an ally?
- Is the bully causing emotional, physical, or social distress?
- Do you feel that an adult needs to intervene?
- If I report it, am I reporting it to get someone in trouble?

If someone is being harmed and you can't stop the bullying yourself you should report it immediately. Protecting the victim is always the right thing to do.

PREVENTING BULLYING

Both parents and school officials have a role in preventing bullying. Parents are important because behavior patterns are learned at home, and because childrearing practices seem to be related to the likelihood that a child will become a bully. However, bullying often occurs in a school setting where teachers and school officials are in a position to do something about it. In addition, schools can offer resources to inform students about the dangers of bullying and ways to prevent it.

The NEA urges parents to talk with their children about their daily experiences as early as possible. This establishes a pattern that can continue when the child starts to attend school. A child who is comfortable talking about his or her day will be more likely to report incidents of bullying at school. Parents also need to be aware of nonverbal indications of bullying such as changes in mood and behavior. The NEA also encourages parents to become familiar with their children's friends and classmates and to volunteer at their school if possible.

How a parent disciplines a child can affect the chances of the child becoming a bully. Parents who hit or yell at their children as a form of discipline teach children that violence and verbal abuse are acceptable ways of dealing with others. Parents should also be aware of the language they use around their children. Casually using racial or ethnic slurs for certain groups of people communicates disrespect for others that children may imitate.

Children who suffer from bullying at school should speak to a teacher or other authority figure. Faculty members are often unaware of problems with bullying, so victims need to alert them when bullying occurs. A child who suffers from bullying should also tell his or her parents. Victims of bullying may have difficulty talking about what happened because of shame or embarrassment. However, silence is worse because it allows the bully to continue victimizing others.

Schools also have a responsibility to take steps to prevent bullying. ASAP recommends that schools adopt codes of conduct that clearly define the behaviors that will not be tolerated and the punishments for those behaviors. Schools should also offer classes to raise student awareness of bullying and teach cooperation instead of confrontation. Anti-bullying programs should include antiviolence, antiracist, and antisexist messages as well. Teachers should praise students for positive social behaviors and reward students who practice cooperative behaviors. These and other activities such as volunteer programs, can help motivate students to act in nonaggressive and helpful ways and reduce the likelihood that they will engage in bullying.

See also: Abusers, Common Traits of; Rehabilitation and Treatment

FURTHER READING

Coloroso, Barbara. *The Bully, the Bullied, and the Bystander: From Preschool to High School—How Parents and Teachers Can Help Break the Cycle of Violence.* New York: HarperResource, 2004.

Elias, Maurice J., and Joseph E. Zins. *Bullying, Peer Harassment, and Vicitmization in the Schools: The Next Generation of Prevention.* Binghamton, NY: Haworth Press, 2004.

Garrett, Anne G. *Bullying in American Schools: Causes, Preventions, Interventions.* Jefferson, NC: McFarland and Company, 2003.

Olweus, Dan. *Bullying at School: What We Know and What We Can Do.* London: Blackwell Publishers, 1993.

■ CHILD ABUSE

The use of physical, emotional, or verbal violence to control the behavior of a child. The Child Abuse Prevention and Treatment Act of 1996 defines child abuse as "any recent act or failure to act, on the part of a parent or caretaker, which results in death, serious physical or emotional harm, sexual abuse or exploitation, or an act or failure to act which presents an imminent risk or serious harm." According to this definition, only parents or caregivers commit child abuse or **neglect** (a failure to take care of a child's physical or emotional needs). A **caregiver** is a person who is responsible for a child's welfare. One of the deep tragedies related to child abuse is the fact that it is committed by those entrusted with the victim's welfare.

DISCIPLINE, ABUSE, AND NEGLECT

Parents who abuse their children often deny that they are abusive. They protest that they have the right to punish their children as they see fit. They say they are disciplining, not abusing. Is some hitting acceptable? Are there good, constructive uses of violence? Where does one draw the line between spanking a child and abuse?

Child experts generally agree that hitting is unacceptable in any relationship. They point out that when a parent or caregiver hits a child, it is considered normal and within the parent's rights; yet in most other situations, it is considered assault, a crime. Those who oppose **corporal punishment** believe that children are the most vulnerable and least protected population.

What is the difference between discipline and abuse? The word *discipline* comes from a Latin word meaning "to teach." According to

Professor Charles Lindquist of California's Fullerton State University, discipline is designed to help teach children control and change their behavior. Its aim is to encourage moral, physical, and intellectual development and a sense of responsibility. Discipline teaches children proper behavior—not because they fear punishment, but because they have learned standards modeled by parents and caregivers. Discipline helps children to become self-reliant and encourages self-confidence and a positive self-image.

Abuse, by contrast, is really not about the child. It is a way for parents or other caregivers to satisfy their own needs or express their feelings. Any improvement in a child's behavior gained through abuse typically is short-lived. The child is likely later to express the hatred and hostility learned from his or her parents in other situations. Rather than fostering a positive self-image, abuse damages the self-esteem of both parents and children.

To some parents, punishment and discipline are the same thing. While the difference between the two seems to be a fine line to some parents and experts, they are very different. Discipline teaches, while abuse harms. Discipline is used to help a child learn; abuse is used to control and even hurt the child.

The term *abuse* implies that the parent or caregiver plays an active role in mistreating a child. However, not all forms of child abuse involve acts such as beating or **verbal abuse**. The media is full of stories of small children who have been left alone while the parents go out. Other equally sensational stories tell of children locked in closets and left for days, dirty and hungry. These are all instances of **neglect**. Physical neglect includes the failure to provide adequate food, clothing or shelter. Emotional neglect is the failure to give love, nurturing, support, or guidance. Neglect can be as damaging as abuse and can lead to the same negative outcomes, both physically and psychologically.

Fact Or Fiction?

Sticks and stones may break my bones, but words will never hurt me.

Fact: Words can leave permanent scars and sometimes the wounds never heal. When the attacks come from one's parents, the damage is even more severe. They may tell a child, "You're stupid, worthless, ugly, and no good. You'll never amount to anything. I wish you were never born. You are nothing but problems." What does one do when he or she hears those words from the people one is expected to trust, believe, and depend on above all others?

Many kids give themselves those same messages. They come to believe those messages. Their self-esteem is shattered. They have no confidence. They think of themselves as failures. It takes a lot of work to overcome those put-downs and insults. But even when they think they have dealt with it, they are constantly fighting the doubts. The saying should be, "Sticks and stones can break my bones, but words just keep on hurting."

CAUSES OF CHILD ABUSE

There is no single cause of child abuse, but research has identified factors that make some people more likely than others to abuse their children. Some of these causes stem from personality traits of the abuser, such as an inability to deal with frustration; others are related to external circumstances such as poverty or single parenthood. Family influences also seem to play a significant role in determining whether someone is likely to become a child abuser.

Studies have shown that people who were abused or who witnessed abuse as children are more likely to become child abusers as adults. In 1993, the *American Journal of Orthopsychiatry* published a study that found a significant percentage of men who were abusive at home had witnessed domestic abuse as children. A 1984 article in the *Journal of Marriage and the Family* found that witnessing violence between one's parents as a child was even more closely related to the likelihood of later abusive behavior than actually suffering child abuse. Child abuse is also more likely in homes where **domestic partner abuse** is occurring. Some of the same traits that lead husbands or boyfriends to batter their partners, such as an inability to control their temper or a need to control others around them, also make them more likely to batter their children.

According to the *1999 National Victim Assistance Academy*, abusers do not know how to express feelings such as anger, frustration, or guilt appropriately. Child abusers often suffer from an inability to control their impulses or deal with frustrations, resulting in violent explosions of temper if they are frustrated by something a child says or does.

In its 2002 *World Report on Health and Violence*, the World Health Organization (WHO) suggests that many child abusers are poorly informed about effective parenting strategies. They do not understand that children at different ages have different needs and capabilities. Abusive parents may wrongly assume that a child is more competent than he or she actually is, or that the child always understands what the parent expects. Basing parenting strategies on such false assumptions can lead to failure and cause the parents to strike out at their children.

Age, marital status, and family income are also important factors in child abuse and neglect. WHO reports that parents who are young, poor, unemployed, and/or single are at greatest risk of abusing their children. This conclusion is borne out by WHO's finding that single mothers commit more child abuse in the United States than any other group.

WHO COMMITS CHILD ABUSE?

Parents commit the overwhelming majority of child abuse violations in the United States. According to the Department of Health and Human Services' Administration for Children and Families (ACF), in 2002 parents were responsible for over 80 percent of all child abuse. The parent most likely to batter a child is the mother. The ACF reported that mothers acting alone committed 40.3 percent of all child abuse violations in 2002. The mother and father together were responsible for a further 18 percent of all child abuse, and the mother together with someone other than the father committed 5.4 percent of child abuse violations. In all, mothers were involved in almost two of every three cases of child abuse.

By contrast, 19.1 percent of reported child abuse cases involved a father acting alone. Fathers, alone or in combination with the mother or another person, committed 38.1 percent of all acts of child abuse. Non-parental guardians (siblings, other family members, babysitters, or guardians) were responsible for about 13 percent of child abuse cases. In just over 3 percent of the cases, the perpetrator was unknown.

FREQUENCY OF CHILD ABUSE

According to the ACF, child protective services agencies in the United States received some 2.6 million reports of abuse concerning 4.5 million children in 2002. The ACF investigated two-thirds of those reports and an estimated 896,000 children were found to be victims of abuse or neglect.

Neglect was the most frequently reported violation, accounting for about 60 percent of the cases. About 20 percent of the children

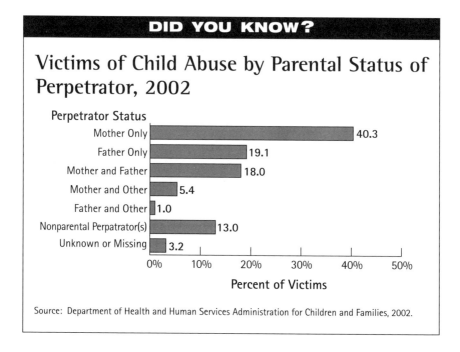

DID YOU KNOW?

Victims of Child Abuse by Parental Status of Perpetrator, 2002

Perpetrator Status

Mother Only	40.3
Father Only	19.1
Mother and Father	18.0
Mother and Other	5.4
Father and Other	1.0
Nonparental Perpatrator(s)	13.0
Unknown or Missing	3.2

0%   10%   20%   30%   40%   50%

Percent of Victims

Source: Department of Health and Human Services Administration for Children and Families, 2002.

reporting abuse were physically abused, and another 10 percent were sexually abused. About 7 percent were victims of **emotional abuse,** which includes criticizing, rejecting, or failing to provide nurturing. Girls are slightly more likely than boys to be abused or neglected, but they are four times as likely to be sexually abused.

The rate of child abuse in the United States in 2002 was 12.3 violations per 1,000 children. Children of all ages are abused or neglected, but very young children are most at risk—the rate among children from birth to three years of age was 16 per 1,000. Among ethnic groups, American Indian and Alaskan Native children suffered the highest rate of abuse (21.7 per 1,000), followed by African-American children (20.2 per thousand). White children experienced the lowest rate of abuse at 10.7 cases per 1,000 children.

In 2002, an estimated 1,400 children in the United States died of abuse or neglect. Of these victims, 76 percent were three years or younger, 12 percent were aged four to seven years, 6 percent were aged eight to 11 years, and another 6 percent were aged 12 to 17 years. Infant boys were most likely to be killed, with a fatality rate of 19 deaths per 100,000. The rate for infant girls was 12 deaths per 100,000. About a third of all child fatalities were due to neglect. Other significant causes of child death were **physical abuse** and sexual abuse (the use of sex to control the actions or behaviors of another person).

EFFECTS OF CHILD ABUSE

Child abuse clearly takes a terrible physical toll each year. However, long after the physical injuries have healed, abused children are at risk of serious emotional problems and developmental difficulties. In 1999, Great Britain's Royal College of Physicians published a leaflet titled "Child Abuse and Neglect: The Emotional Effects." It outlined the college's findings about the long-term psychological harm done to children of abuse. According to the leaflet, physically abused children may show the following emotional and behavioral symptoms:

- Developing poor self-esteem
- Becoming passive and lacking initiative
- Throwing temper tantrums
- Becoming aggressive or abusive themselves (bullying other children)
- Having difficulty forming close friendships
- Lying, stealing, or skipping school
- Getting into trouble with the police

In addition, abused children often show developmental problems, including:

- Delays in learning to walk or talk
- Slower than normal growth
- Difficulty concentrating in school
- Poor school performance

If you know someone who shows several of these symptoms, it is possible that person may be the victim of abuse. If the person is a friend, perhaps he or she would be willing to talk to you about the problem. If not, encourage him or her to talk to a counselor or a social services agency. The most important first step for the victim is to get out of the abusive situation.

TEENS SPEAK

I've Had Lots of Injuries but Only Went to the Hospital If I Broke a "Bone"

I've broken a few bones, but my father took me to different hospitals each time so the doctors wouldn't have a record of it. The doctors at one hospital got suspicious when I broke my collarbone, but my father had an explanation—I fell off the deck. I was only nine. I was scared to tell the truth—that he had pushed me and I fell down the stairs—because I thought he would hurt me more. I loved him and didn't want to get him into trouble. He worked hard to support us. He was just really stressed out. Besides, what would we do if he went to jail?

My sixth grade teacher started asking questions when I came in with bruises and a black eye. The worst thing was that I had also lost a front tooth. I tried to tell her the "official" story about a run-in with a door, but I couldn't stop crying and told her the real story about a run-in with my father instead. She had to report him.

A woman from social services took my brother and me to a shelter, away from my stepmother and father. We were in foster care for a while, but we went back home a few months later. My father said he had counseling and learned how to deal with his frustration better. We still get regular visits from social services to check on how we're doing. My father still has a temper, but he doesn't take it out on us anymore.

THE LAW AND CHILD ABUSE

People in some professions are required by law to report suspected child abuse or neglect to child protective or social services departments. These people include doctors, dentists, social service workers, childcare workers, police, school officials and teachers, nurses, and mental health professionals.

Sometimes neighbors, friends, or relatives call the authorities to report suspected abuse. Anyone who suspects that abuse is occurring should call a child protective department. If one is reluctant to become involved, one can leave an anonymous report. There are also national and local reporting hotlines. Child Protective Services or another local government social services agency will investigate to see if there are grounds for the accusation. If law enforcement and social services have some proof of abuse, they can take several actions. They may remove the children from the home and place them in temporary foster care until the case can be investigated more thoroughly. In some cases, parents may lose their rights to custody of the children, who may be placed in long-term foster care or with relatives. A parent may even be jailed if the abuse is severe. Above anything else, the safety and welfare of children are the priority.

Legal and child-welfare authorities want to keep families together if it is at all possible to do so. Social services agencies work with parents or guardians to address the problems that lead to the abuse and teach them better parenting and coping skills. If drinking or drugs are involved, the parents will be ordered to attend a rehabilitation program and avoid using those substances in the future. Some critics, however, say that children are too often returned to their homes only to endure more abuse.

If children are in serious immediate danger or have been left alone by their parents or guardians, a police officer, a doctor, or a child services officer can have them taken into protective custody. The children may be placed in foster care until the courts decide whether they should return to their homes, be placed with relatives, or remain in foster care on a long-term basis.

The system of placing children in foster care or with relatives is often criticized. Critics claim that children are separated from their brothers and sisters, and that they are moved from foster family to foster family and have little stability. In some cases, children are sent to live with relatives whose backgrounds have not been checked for abuse. They also may be taken from stable foster homes and returned to their parents before the problems at home have been corrected.

Charges of child abuse place law enforcement and child-welfare workers in a difficult position. The state wants to protect children from harm, but it is also reluctant to break up families. While child-welfare agencies try to do what is best for the child and the family, they often struggle with a lack of personnel and funding. These considerations make preventing child abuse and dealing with its aftermath a major challenge to law enforcement and social services agencies throughout the United States.

Q & A

Question: Will I get my parents in trouble if I tell my teacher that they used to hurt me and now they are hitting my little brother?

Answer: You are right to worry about your brother's safety (and your own). If you tell your teacher, she will have to report it to the authorities. She is one of the people required by law to report child abuse. It may seem that you are getting your parents into trouble, but you are really getting your brother and yourself out of harm's way. Be aware, however, that you and your brother may be taken to live somewhere else to protect you both. Parents who have been reported may become angrier and more violent. They may blame you for breaking the silence about their behavior. If you are scared about what will happen, talk to a trusted adult first, one who is not required to report child abuse to legal authorities. He or she can help you sort out your options.

See also: Abuse in Society; Abuse, Witnesses of; Child Sexual Abuse; Legal Intervention; Post-traumatic Stress Disorder and Abuse; Psychological Abuse

FURTHER READING

American Prosecutors Research Institute. *Investigation and Prosecution of Child Abuse.* Thousand Oaks, CA: Sage Publications, 2003.

Crosson-Tower, Cynthia. *Understanding Child Abuse and Neglect, Fifth Edition.* Boston: Allyn and Bacon, 2001.

Sagatun, Inger, and Leonard Edwards. *Child Abuse and the Legal System.* Belmont, CA: Wadsworth Publishing Company, 1995.

Matthews, Dawn D. *Child Abuse Sourcebook: Basic Consumer Health Information about the Physical, Sexual, and Emotional Abuse of Children.* Detroit: Omnigraphics, 2004.

■ CHILD SEXUAL ABUSE

The use of sexual behavior as a way to control the actions or behaviors of a child. Sexual abuse of children is a complex problem that has lasting effects on its victims. The true extent of the problem is not known because so many victims keep quiet about it. Even when child sexual abuse is reported, it is often difficult for the authorities to prove it happened. If there is no witness or physical sign of abuse, it can become a matter of taking the word of the child or the word of the adult. Some victims may wait until adulthood to reveal the abuse they suffered. Others never report it.

DEFINING CHILD SEXUAL ABUSE

Sexual activity includes both physical touching and acts that do not involve contact with the child. Physical acts include:

- Sexually touching a child
- Forcing a child to sexually touch an adult
- Stripping a child for spanking
- Engaging in oral, vaginal, or anal intercourse with a child
- Forcing a child to engage in prostitution

Noncontact acts that are considered sexual abuse include:

- Taking pornographic pictures of a child
- Showing pornography to a child
- Talking to a child in a sexual manner
- Exposing oneself to a child
- **Verbal abuse** or **emotional abuse** of a sexual nature
- Touching oneself in front of a child
- "Peeping" on a child who is dressing or showering

In most states, certain conditions must apply before an act can be considered child sexual abuse. The child must be young enough that he or she is considered incapable of consenting to the act. Many states require that there be a minimum age difference between the victim and the offender. In Texas, for example, the offender must be at least three years older than the victim for an act to be considered child sexual abuse. Any case involving sexual activity between an adult and a **juvenile**, or between an older teen and a young child, would be considered child sexual abuse.

Fact Or Fiction?

Most child molesters are only attracted to children and are not capable of having sexual relationships with adults.

Fact: Most child molesters fall into one of two categories. About 35 per cent are attracted to children as their primary sexual interest. They are called fixated child molesters, or pedophiles. Most child molesters—about

65 percent—are called regressive offenders. They are primarily interested in adults. However, if the opportunity presents itself, they may "regress" and seek sex and emotional comfort from a child. Some are under the influence of drugs or alcohol, which helps to lower their inhibitions. Even so, they would not commit child sexual abuse unless they already had those fantasies or desires.

RATES OF ABUSE

Experts disagree about the extent of child sexual abuse in the United States but agree that it is a widespread problem. According to the National Center for Post-Traumatic Stress Disorder (NCPTSD), about 10 percent of all boys in the United States—and as many as 25 percent of all girls—are sexually abused. In the 2001 article "Sexual Abuse of Children," researcher Renee Dominguez reported that up to 25 percent of boys and 33 percent of girls have been victims of sexual abuse. The Department of Justice found that 1.8 million children between the ages of 12 and 17 were sexually abused in 1997.

According to Dominguez, girls are far more likely to be victimized than boys. They are twice as likely to be victims of sexual abuse as children, and eight times as likely as boys to be sexually abused as adolescents. In addition, 62 percent of all forcible rape occurs before the age of 18, and almost half of that figure (30 percent) occurs before age 11.

Who commits child sexual abuse?

Sexual abuse can be particularly confusing and damaging to children because the victims usually know and trust their abusers. According to the NCPTSD, someone the victim knows commits some 90 percent of all child sexual abuse. About 60 percent of the perpetrators or abusers are people who are not related to the child. They include friends, neighbors, baby-sitters, and, even on occasion, teachers, counselors, or clergy. Relatives of the victim are responsible for about 30 percent of all child sexual abuse. Men commit the vast majority of child abuse, but women are involved in 14 percent of cases of abuse against boys and 6 percent of cases of abuse against girls.

The idea that most child abusers are "dirty old men" hanging out on street corners is a myth. Only about 10 percent of all child abuse is committed by strangers. It is the sense of familiarity and trust that exists between the child and his abuser that allows sexual abuse to occur. It is also this aspect of the abuse—the fact that it is committed by a trusted authority figure—that can make it so damaging.

TEENS SPEAK

I Asked Him to Stop, But He Wouldn't

When I was about nine years old, my parents got a divorce. I missed my father a lot. So did my eight-year-old brother. Just after that, my mother started dating David. He moved in with us about a year later. He was nice to us before he moved in, and he was really nice for the first few months he lived with us. He played with us and he tucked us in at night. I felt close to him, even though he wasn't my real father, but then he started touching me all over under the covers. He threatened to leave us if I told my mother or my real father. I didn't like what he was doing, but I didn't want him to leave. I liked him, and my brother and mother seemed happier with him in the house.

This went on for years. He got even more touchy with me and wanted me to touch him too. I didn't like it, and I didn't like to be near him anymore. Sometimes I wished he would go away, but on the other hand, he treated me like I was so special. I didn't say anything and I tried to pretend for my mother and brother that everything was okay. But sometimes I felt so angry and I didn't really know why.

Then, when I was 13, we learned about sexual abuse in health class. I knew right away that was what was happening with David. The teacher said to tell an adult if it was happening. I went to her after class and told her I thought I was being abused. She said that she would have to report it, and she told me to tell my mother.

My mom got hysterical. Some people came and investigated. David can't live with us anymore, and my brother is mad at me. At first I wished I hadn't said anything. I thought to myself that I should have just lived with what was happening until I was old enough to go away to school. I think I felt worse about the trouble I had caused than I did about what David was doing to me.

I told my health teacher how bad things were at home. She helped our family get counseling. The counselor helped us all understand that I wasn't the person who was at fault. David had caused the problems, not me. I still don't quite understand David. He seemed really happy with my mother. Maybe some day I'll talk to him. I'll tell him how much he hurt me. And I'll ask him why.

Adolescents who abuse

Children abuse each other, too, but there is a big difference between two six-year-olds playing doctor and a teenaged baby-sitter touching a toddler's genitals. To identify abuse by a juvenile, several factors are important: the age, the power or force used (either physical or emotional force), and the younger child's ability to understand what is happening. If a child overpowers another through age, size, or threats, it is abuse. If one child understands what is happening and the other doesn't, that is also abuse.

A 1997 study published in the journal *Pediatrics* found that 4.8 percent of male adolescents and 1.3 percent of female adolescents said they had forced someone into a sexual act. The study, "Adolescent Sexual Aggression: Risk and Protective Factors," found that certain behaviors—including gang membership and use of alcohol, illicit drugs, or steroids—increased a teen's chances of becoming a sexual abuser. Having lots of idle free time also seemed to be a risk factor for committing sexual abuse. Male teens who said they "hung out" more than 40 hours a week were more likely to have forced someone into a sexual act.

Exposure to family violence seems to be strongly related to sexual abuse by adolescents. Male youths who had witnessed or been the victims of family violence were twice as likely to child commit sexual abuse as those with no family history of abuse. A 1996 study reported in the *Journal of the American Academy of Child and Adolescent Psychiatry*, "Trends in a National Sample of Sexually Abusive Youth," studied 1,600 male youths arrested for sexual offenses and found that 42 percent had been physically abused. A further 39 percent had been sexually abused and 63 percent had witnessed family violence. Interestingly, neither being physically abused nor witnessing family violence made female teens more likely to become sexually abusive.

What factors may reduce the chances of a child growing up to be sexually abusive toward other children? Males who have strong relationships with parents, family, and friends are less likely to become sexual abusers. Having close ties with adults in the community through organizations such as schools and religious groups also offers protection against becoming an abuser. Female teens who perform well academically are at less risk than their peers who are not doing as well at school.

SIGNS OF ABUSE

One of the most frustrating aspects of child abuse is that there is often little or no clear evidence that abuse has occurred. In addition, children do not usually speak directly about the sexual abuse. They may not have the knowledge, understanding, or language to tell accurately what has happened. They may be too embarrassed or ashamed. If the abuser is someone close to the family, the child may feel guilty about getting that person into trouble. They may even blame themselves for the abuse. In many cases, a child may also fear that revealing the abuse will bring even worse consequences. Perhaps the child will not be believed, and the abuser may retaliate against the child.

There are, however, certain signs that strongly suggest that a child has been sexually abused. Physical clues include genital or rectal pain or bleeding, genital warts and other **sexually transmitted diseases** (STDs), **HIV**, and even pregnancy. Emotional and behavioral clues to sexual abuse are more difficult to spot. The NCPTSD reports that, although certain symptoms such as low self-esteem or behavior problems are characteristic of sexual abuse victims; different victims show different combinations of symptoms.

EFFECTS OF ABUSE

The most common psychological effect of child sexual abuse is **post-traumatic stress disorder,** or PTSD. PTSD is a severe response to a traumatic event during which the child may reenact or reexperience the abuse. At the other extreme, the child may avoid anything that reminds him or her of the abuse. For example, the child may refuse to go to school or church if the abuse took place there. Other symptoms associated with PTSD that frequently occur as a result of sexual abuse include:

- Behavior problems
- Poor self-esteem
- Acting out sexually

- Depression

- Anxiety

- Self-mutilation or attempted suicide

Recent research has shown that child sexual abuse can have health consequences that last into adulthood. According to researcher Renee Dominguez, these effects can include depression, anxiety, sexual disorders, and substance abuse. Adult females who were sexually abused as children are twice as likely to commit suicide as those who were not abused. Victims of childhood sexual abuse are also four times more likely to develop mental disorders as adults and three times more likely to become substance abusers.

Some factors can reduce the seriousness of the long-term effects of child sexual abuse. Dominguez reports that the long–term effects of sexual abuse depend upon the age of the child, how long the abuse went on, how often it occurred, the amount of force used, and the relationship of the abuser to the child. If the abuse occurred over a long period of time, or the abuser was a parent or close family member, the effects are usually more severe. Children with lower self-esteem usually suffer worse than those with a more positive self-image.

A child who is able to tell a trusted adult about the abuse is less likely to suffer severe long-term problems. Having a close and supportive family environment also helps reduce the impact of abuse. A parent's reaction to the abuse also has an effect on the way the child reacts. The more shock, anger, or distress the parent expresses upon hearing of the abuse, the more negatively the incident will affect the child. Receiving the news in a concerned but calm manner will do more to reassure the child and lessen the impact of the abuse.

RESPONDING TO CHILD SEXUAL ABUSE

A child shows considerable courage when he or she tells someone about sexual abuse, especially if the abuser is a relative, teacher, or other important person in his or her life. It is important for family members to listen to the child and take the accusations seriously, even if the accused person is a trusted friend or relative. Parents are often understandably reluctant to believe that Uncle George or Cousin Tim or even Grandpa is hurting their child. The abuser will usually deny the abuse, and some parents may be willing to accept the word of the adult over the child.

Reporting child sexual abuse

Many adults, including parents, are reluctant to report sexual abuse for fear that it will be traumatic for the child. However, children need to feel that adults are keeping them safe. Trying to take care of the abuse within the family may not ensure safety. Failing to report abuse also leaves other children at risk of abuse. Not only do parents have a moral obligation to investigate a child's claims of abuse, they also have a legal obligation to do so. In Texas, for example, child abuse charges can be filed against a parent who is aware of child sexual abuse but fails to report it.

Other adults—including teachers, doctors, and mental health professionals—are also legally required to report child sexual abuse. Such individuals are called **mandated adults** because they have a mandate (legal requirement) to report abuse. However, anyone can report suspected abuse. Children and teens can even call the authorities themselves.

Q & A

Question: I told my parents about being sexually abused. Is that enough or should I go for counseling?

Answer: Telling your parents is a good first step, but you should follow it up by talking to a counselor. A trained counselor will help you deal with many of your fears about your own sexuality, what other people will think if they know about the abuse, and how to take charge of your own body. A counselor will help you become more comfortable with yourself and regain trust in others. He or she will help you see that it was not your fault and that it has happened to other teens. Even if you have a close relationship with your parents or another adult, it can be very helpful to talk to someone who can be more objective and not get emotional when you talk about your feelings.

Investigating and prosecuting abuse

Every state has agencies to investigate physical and sexual abuse of children. If the abuser is the child's caregiver or lives in the same home, a child protection agency (a government agency responsible for dealing with cases of child abuse) investigates. If the abuser is a stranger, neighbor, or some other person not living with the child, the police will investigate. Any report of child abuse, sexual or physical, is supposed to be investigated. For young children or children who are shy about talking, the interviewer may use puppets, or anatomically correct dolls or drawings, to determine what happened. For toddlers or babies, the investigator must rely on information from a doctor and parents. The alleged abuser is also interviewed.

The prosecutor or district attorney decides if there is enough evidence to prosecute the accused abuser. If the prosecutors do not take cases to trial, it does not mean they don't believe that abuse occurred. They may have determined that the case is too difficult to prove because the child is too young to testify, or that there is not enough medical evidence to prove abuse. This may leave parents frustrated and angry, and older children confused. "Why didn't they believe me?" the child might ask.

When charges are brought against an alleged abuser, the victim and family can be in for a long legal process. It can be especially difficult if a child must testify against a parent or other close relative. Dominguez reports that a child may reexperience the trauma of the sexual abuse. The victim is often interviewed repeatedly about the incident and must retell the story again and again. About 95 percent of victims say they are afraid to testify in court against their abusers. Many fear the perpetrator will try to get back at them for testifying. Others say they fear being sent to jail, having to prove that they are innocent, or that they will be punished for making a mistake when testifying. By being aware of these potential difficulties, parents can make the reporting and trial process easier for children to understand and accept.

See also: Abuse, Witnesses of; Alcohol, Drugs, and Abuse; Child Abuse; Domestic Partner Abuse; Men and Abuse; Women and Abuse

FURTHER READING

Bagley, Christopher, Kanka Mallick, and the Center for Evaluative and Developmental Research. *Child Sexual Abuse and Adult Offenders: New Theory and Research.* Williston, VT: Ashgate Publishing Company, 1999.

Conte, John R. *Critical Issues in Child Sexual Abuse: Historical, Legal, and Psychological Perspectives.* Thousand Oaks, CA: Sage Publications, 2002.

Elliott, Michelle. *Female Sexual Abuse of Children.* New York: Guilford Publications, 1994.

Erooga, Marcus, and Helen C. Masson. *Children and Young People Who Sexually Abuse Others: Challenges and Responses.* London: Routledge, 1999.

Van Dam, Carla. *Identifying Child Molesters: Preventing Child Sexual Abuse by Recognizing the Patterns of the Offenders.* London: Haworth Press, 2001.

■ DATING ABUSE

Any hurtful or unwanted physical, sexual, verbal, or emotional act inflicted by a casual or intimate dating partner. Like child abuse and domestic partner abuse, dating abuse covers a wide range of actions, including insults, threats, false accusations, and controlling behavior as well as physical assault and rape. Dating abuse is shockingly common in the United States, and a great deal of it occurs between teens. Teen dating abuse is particularly troubling, because it may signal the beginning of a pattern of abuse that can persist into adulthood.

TEENS SPEAK

I Was So Happy to Find Someone Else in My School Who Was a Lesbian

Before I met Jody, I was having a really tough time since my friends and family didn't know about my sexual orientation. Jody and I got along really well at first. Then I guess I got a little possessive. It's just that I didn't want to lose her. She wasn't "out" to her friends but she spent a lot of time with them. I was afraid she would get a crush on this one girl in particular. Her other friends thought we were just friends, so they didn't seem to understand why Jody was hanging out with me instead of them. I felt like they were trying to pull her away from me.

I told her I didn't want her to spend time with them. She knew that I had a bad temper, because I once threw a book at her and another time I pushed her, but we were alone when that happened. When she said she had something else to do after school one day, I got angry and slammed her locker door hard while she was putting her books away. Everyone was looking and she got embarrassed and maybe a little scared and ran down the hallway. Then the gossip started about me being gay and that I had a crush on her. No one knew that she was a lesbian too, so I threatened to "out her" if she didn't keep dating me.

It wasn't that we didn't have fun together. But I scared her, and she said she never knew if or when I was going to go off on her. She finally broke it off. I tried to hang on to her and even threatened to tell her parents that she was gay.

I guess she was scared of me because she told a school counselor. Now I'm glad she did. The counselor hooked me up with a Gay/Lesbian/Bisexual/Transgender/Questioning youth group. She also helped me find a psychologist who works with teens who are abusive toward their partners. Jody may have been the best thing that happened to me.

INCIDENCE OF DATING ABUSE

In her 1988 book *Warning! Dating May Be Hazardous to Your Health*, Claudette McShane, a professor of social work, claims that women in the United States have a 50 percent chance of suffering some type of abuse in a dating relationship. *Getting Free: A Handbook for Women in Abusive Relationships* reports that between 25 and 50 percent of all women who have intimate relationships with men will experience physical abuse in the relationship at least once. Author Ginny NiCarthy, an activist and counselor in the movement to end violence against women, says that an even greater percentage suffer emotional abuse. A 1989 review of research on dating abuse titled "Dating Violence: Prevalence, Context, and Risk Markers" found even higher numbers. The study reported that up to 65 percent of women in dating relationships are victims of physical, sexual, verbal and emotional violence.

Dating abuse happens to women of all ages. Some 25 percent of the eighth- and ninth-grade girls surveyed for the study had suffered nonsexual violence at the hands of a dating partner. Another 8 percent had been the victims of sexual abuse by their partner. In a 2002 survey by the South Boston *Patriot Ledger,* about 20 percent of high school students knew someone who was forced to have sex by a date but did not report the assault to the police.

According to the 1987 article "The Scope of Rape: Incidence and Prevalence of Sexual Aggression and Victimization in a National Sample of Higher Education Students," 27.5 percent of female college students nationwide had experienced rape or attempted rape at least once since age 14. The article points out that only 5 percent of those assaults were reported to police. In 1996 *The Psychology of Women Quarterly* published a survey of sexual abuse among women at a large urban university. Of the more than 1,000 women who responded to the survey, over 50 percent said they had experienced unwanted sex.

These rates of abuse and assault are based on what is reported to interviewers or the police. A large proportion of date abuse is never reported. In his 1993 book *In Love and in Danger*, Barrie Levy estimated that 28 percent of high school girls who have been sexually abused by a date did not tell anyone about the attack. According to the National Center for Injury Prevention and Control (NCIPC), researchers refer to this phenomenon as "hidden rape."

Some studies show that women are more likely than men to be the victims of dating violence. For example, Levy cites figures claiming that women are victims of 91 percent of all assaults committed by a dating partner. In addition, studies in 1983 and 1986 found that girls and women were victims of dating violence twice as often and men. However, two other studies—"Prevalence and Correlates of Physical Aggression during Courtship" and "Courtship Violence: Incidence in a National Sample of Higher Education Students"—suggest that there is little difference in the rates of dating aggression committed by males and females. Those studies found that women most often commit violence to defend themselves from their partners.

When dating violence does occur, there is little question that women suffer the most from its effects. Females experience significantly more injuries from dating violence than do males. According to the Federal Bureau of Investigation, 40 percent of all female murder victims in 1995 were killed by a husband or boyfriend.

CHARACTERISTICS OF ABUSERS AND VICTIMS

Researchers have identified several factors that tend to increase the risks of dating abuse, but most of these risk factors apply to men. In its online report "Dating Violence," the NCIPC, a division of the Centers for Disease Control and Prevention (CDC), summarizes recent research on dating abuse. According to that report, studies have identified the following characteristics of potential abusers:

- Alcohol or drug use. A 1993 article in the *Journal of Sex Education and Therapy* found that 67.5 percent of college males who sexually assaulted their dates had been drinking.
- Witnessing or suffering abuse as a child. Ginny NiCarthy found that some 60 percent of the men she studied were raised in homes where they were battered or witnessed battering.
- Having sexually aggressive **peers**
- Taking "control" roles on a date, including initiating the date, being the driver, or paying for all expenses
- Holding stereotypical ideas about sex roles
- A history of violence

The NCIPC has also noted several characteristics that seem to increase the likelihood of suffering dating abuse. These include:

- Drug or alcohol abuse. Drug and alcohol abuse increases the chances of experiencing dating abuse as well as committing it. Research cited in the NCIPC report showed that both the frequency and seriousness of injuries increase with greater intake of alcohol or drugs by either the abuser or the victim.
- Having friends who were victims. In 1987, a study in the journal *Family Relations* reported that females whose friends were sexually victimized by dates were at greater risk of dating abuse.
- Having a large number of dating partners
- Accepting dating abuse as "normal"
- Having previously been a victim of sexual assault

ATTITUDES TOWARD DATING ABUSE

Some widely held attitudes about the proper roles of men and women, or what kind of behavior is acceptable between partners, contributes significantly to dating abuse. For example, Levy found that 25 to 35 percent of the young people she interviewed who were victims of dating abuse interpreted violence by their partner as an expression of love. In addition, 60 percent of those couples said that the violence had no effect on their relationship. Of the college women Levy surveyed,

70 percent felt that some form of abuse—either physical, sexual, verbal, or emotional—was acceptable in an intimate relationship.

Fact Or Fiction?

If you buy your date dinner and the movie, she owes you sex.

Fact: Your date never owes you anything except a "thank you." Sex is not repayment or some kind of trade-off. You shouldn't ever make your date feel as if she is in your debt. If you take her to dinner and a movie, do it because you want to treat her to a good time, not because you want something from her. If you can't afford dinner and a movie, then talk to her about money, not about sex! (By the way, there is also no rule that says the guy has to pay for the date.)

Attitudes about what kind of dating behavior is and is not acceptable apparently develop at a fairly early age. In the *Patriot Ledger* study of high school students, 15 percent of boys said that it is okay to force a girl to have sex if she initially says yes but later changes her mind. In addition, 20 percent of boys said it was sometimes acceptable to force a girl to have sex if they have been dating steadily and previously had sex. In fact, the more serious or long-term the relationship, the more likely violence is to occur. Levy reports that between 47 and 86 percent of dating violence happens during the serious or "steady" phase of the relationship.

RECOGNIZING A POTENTIAL ABUSER

According to the Cooperative Extension to the University of Nebraska at Lincoln, the earliest forms of violence in a dating relationship typically are intimidation and threats. However, the violence is likely to increase in frequency and seriousness over time. It is therefore extremely important to recognize early signs that suggest a partner may be abusive. Such warning signs include:

- Losing one's temper more often and more easily than seems appropriate
- Abusing alcohol or illegal drugs
- Extreme jealousy

- Anger when a partner does not follow his or her advice or accept his or her opinions

- The expectation that he or she will spend all of their time together or the partner will notify him or her of the partner's whereabouts

- Attempts to control a partner's appearance, including how he or she dresses

- Following a partner to see what he or she is doing and where he or she is going

- Slapping, hitting, or pushing a partner

- Having been physically or verbally abused at home or having parents in an abusive relationship

Q & A

Question: I've heard about something called "date rape drugs." What are date rape drugs and how dangerous are they?

Answer: Date rape drugs are a variety of substances that, when slipped into a drink, can render the victim helpless against sexual assault.

The most common date rape drug is flunitrazepam, or Rohypnol, also known as "roofies." Rohypnol is a prescription drug used by physicians to treat insomnia and to prepare patients for anesthesia before an operation. Although legal in Europe, it cannot be produced or sold legally in the United States. However, it is smuggled into the United States through the mail and delivery services.

In most cases, Rohypnol is slipped into an alcoholic beverage, where its effects combine with the intoxicating effects of the alcohol. The behavioral effects of Rohypnol include drowsiness, dizziness, confusion, and memory impairment. Not only is the victim defenseless against sexual assault, but Rohypnol also makes it very difficult to remember what happened under the influence of the drug. Many girls and women report awakening and realizing they have been assaulted, but they have no memory of the crime. Since the drug is colorless and odorless, you may have no warning you have been drugged until it is too late.

There are steps you can take to avoid being the victim of a date rape drug. These include:

- Don't accept drinks from someone you don't know or trust

- Only accept drinks in unopened containers

- Don't leave your drink unattended, even for a few minutes

The Nebraska Cooperative Extension suggests taking the following steps to reduce the chances of becoming a victim of dating abuse:

■ Communicate to your partner your expectations about how he or she will treat you. Use both verbal communication (such as saying "no" to unwanted sexual advances) and nonverbal communication (such as leaving when he or she becomes physically or verbally abusive).

■ Refuse to be passive or to allow your partner to take the "control" roles in your relationship. Tell and show your partner that he or she cannot always be in charge.

■ Trust your intuition. If you feel that something is not right in your relationship do not simply dismiss the feeling.

DEALING WITH AND PREVENTING DATING ABUSE

If you or someone you know has been the victim of dating abuse, the Nebraska Cooperative Extension suggests taking the following steps:

■ Report the abuse to someone. Go to a friend, parent, counselor, or law enforcement official. Do not let the abuser get away to assault someone else.

■ Seek medical treatment. Go to a hospital or physician that can treat your injuries and examine you for evidence that can be used in court. Do not shower, bathe, douche, or change clothes beforehand, as doing so may destroy evidence the police need to convict the attacker.

■ Seek counseling. Professional support can be crucial to helping victims understand and deal with what has happened, to reassure them that they were not to blame, and to help them start on the road to recovery. A counselor may also be able to recommend a support group consisting of others who have experienced dating abuse.

In addition to offering suggestions for self-help, the Cooperative Extension also provides advice on preventing dating abuse before it occurs. Suggestions include:

- Assisting community prevention efforts. Help local businesses and community organizations such as churches or the YMCA educate people about the risk factors associated with dating abuse. Encourage groups in the community to initiate such programs.

- Encouraging your school to start a "no violence" campaign that teaches students appropriate dating behavior and effective strategies for resisting unwanted sex.

- Working with your family to identify dysfunctional behavior that can lead to domestic violence.

- Being a role model for appropriate dating behavior. Avoid stereotypical sex-role attitudes and behaviors and encourage your friends to avoid them as well. Model respectful and nonviolent actions and expect the same of others.

- Seeking counseling if you see signs of violence in your family or in a dating relationship.

See also: Alcohol, Drugs, and Abuse; Domestic Partner Abuse: Men and Abuse; Sexual Abuse; Sexual Assault; Women and Abuse

FURTHER READING

Kehner, George, and David J. Triggle. *Date Rape Drugs.* London: Chelsea House Publications, 2004.

Levy, Barrie. *In Love and in Danger: A Teen's Guide to Breaking Free of Abusive Relationships.* New York: Seal Press, 1998.

Lloyd, Sally A., and Beth C. Emory. *The Dark Side of Courtship: Physical and Sexual Aggression.* Thousand Oaks, CA: Sage Publications, 1999.

Sanders, Susan M. *Teen Dating Abuse: The Invisible Peril.* New York: Peter Lang Publishing, 2003.

Wolfe, David A., Christine Wekerle, and Katrina Scott. *Alternatives to Violence: Empowering Youth to Develop Healthy Relationships.* Thousand Oaks, CA: Sage Publications, 1998.

■ DEPRESSION AND ABUSE

See: Abuse, Theories of; Post-traumatic Stress Disorder; Psychological Abuse

■ DOMESTIC PARTNER ABUSE

The use of physical, emotional, or verbal violence to control a domestic partner. A domestic partner is a person (not necessarily a spouse) with whom one lives and shares a long-term sexual relationship. Domestic partners include couples living together in heterosexual, lesbian, or gay relationships. Domestic partner abuse has many names: spousal abuse, domestic abuse, domestic assault, wife beating, mate beating, or **battering**.

The terms *domestic abuse, domestic partner abuse*, and *battering* are used interchangeably. Battering is a pattern of abuse that occurs over a period of time. While domestic abuse can be a single or one-time incident, it usually escalates (gets worse and more frequent over time). When a person is repeatedly abused, he or she is said to have been **battered**.

DEFINITIONS OF DOMESTIC PARTNER ABUSE

The legal definition of domestic abuse is very narrow and focuses on physical danger or injury. Although legal definitions vary from state to state, most are similar to the following definition used in a Florida law:

'Domestic violence' means any assault, aggravated assault, battery, aggravated battery, sexual assault, sexual battery, stalking, aggravated stalking, kidnapping, false imprisonment, or any criminal offense resulting in physical injury or death of one family or household member by another who is or was residing in the same single dwelling unit."

Mental health experts define abusive behavior in broader terms. They consider abuse any behavior that controls or exerts power over another person. Thus, partner abuse is not simply assault caused by frustration or anger. Instead, it arises from the desire of an individual to limit a spouse or partner's (or former spouse or partner's) freedom.

The list of behaviors that psychologists consider domestic abuse is large. It includes **verbal abuse** such as shouting, threats of violence, threats of abandonment, false accusations, and insults. Domestic abuse can take the form of emotional violence such as withholding affection, isolating a partner from outside social contact, or cheating on one's spouse. A partner may also engage in economic abuse such as taking complete control of finances and making the other partner financially dependent. Of course, abuse also includes physical assaults such as punching, kicking, or slapping, as well as sexual assault. Not all of these forms of abuse are criminal acts, but all serve to reinforce the abuser's control over the victim.

THE CYCLE OF ABUSE

Battering is not an isolated act of abuse now and then. It is a pattern of abuse used to control another person. Although the abusive partner may claim that he or she just lost his or her temper, was letting off steam, or just couldn't help it, those are excuses. If the batterer is able to keep his or her temper in check with other people, or even with his or her partner when they are out in public, then he does have the ability to control abusive actions.

Psychologists talk about a common pattern called the "cycle of violence." This theory was first outlined by Lenore Walker in her 1979 book *The Battered Woman*. Walker's theory focuses on the dynamics between battered women and male abusers. She argues that battering often occurs in a pattern that has three phases: the tension-building stage, the battering stage, and a makeup period called "the honeymoon phase."

During the buildup stage, the tension mounts. The abuser complains, calls the victim names, makes accusations, and blames the partner for all sorts of irritations. The victim is "walking on eggshells" and trying to do anything possible to avoid setting off the abuser's inevitable explosion.

The second stage is the explosion. No matter how much the partner tries to please the abuser, eventually his anger and rage boil over and he attacks her—verbally, emotionally, physically or all three. This is a brief and dangerous time lasting a few minutes to nearly 24 hours.

The third stage is the honeymoon. This is the quiet after the storm. The abuser is sorry for his rage. He behaves lovingly and promises it will never happen again. The victim chooses to believe that this loving person is the "real" partner, the person she fell in love with. She decides to give him another chance. This phase keeps her in the relationship because she is sure that this time he will change; this time he was so violent he even scared himself. However, the cycle of violence not only continues but also increases in intensity and frequency. It will often continue until the woman gets out—or is killed.

Fact Or Fiction?

Victims must like being abused; otherwise they'd leave.

Fact: Many people blame the victims for not leaving or think there is something wrong with them, but there are many barriers to leaving. In many cases it is dangerous to leave. The abuser could become more violent if the victim tries to leave. Leaving can also mean living in fear of losing child custody, losing financial support, and being harassed at work by the abuser. The victim's friends and family may not provide emotional support for leaving. The victim also may continue to hope that the abuser will change. The cycle of abuse is often what keeps a victim in an abusive relationship.

RATES OF ABUSE

Many people mistakenly believe that strangers commit most acts of violence in the United States. The sad fact is that the majority of violence occurs in the very relationships in which people should feel most safe and loved. The people who often do the most harm are people known to the victims and trusted by them. Violence by a partner is one of the most common and dangerous types of abuse. Former Secretary of Health and Human Services Donna Shalala called domestic partner abuse "terrorism in the home."

According to a 2000 analysis of data about domestic abuse by the Bureau of Justice Statistics (BJS), just over one million incidents of domestic abuse were reported in 1998. The report, *Violence by Intimates: Analysis of Data on Crimes by Current or Former Spouses, Boyfriends, and Girlfriends*, showed that domestic partner abuse can continue even after a relationship has ended.

Many people think that male partners commit most domestic abuse, but research has questioned that assumption. A 1990 study titled "Physical Violence in American Families: Risk Factors and Adaptations to Violence in Families" suggested that females commit domestic abuse almost as often as men. However, a 1992 article in the journal *Social Problems*, found that most of the instances in which women committed domestic violence were cases of self-defense. In some instances, the violence was an immediate reaction to violence by a partner. In others, women who had suffered abuse over a long period struck back at their abusers.

Although the rate of abuse may be similar for women and men, women report abuse much more frequently than men. The BJS found that women reported domestic abuse at five times the rate men did. In 1998 women were reported as victims in 876,340 cases of abuse in the United States, while men were victims in 157,330 reports. Domestic abuse accounts for 22 percent of all violent crime against women, but only 3 percent of violent crime against men.

As tragic as these numbers are, they actually represent an improvement in recent years. In 1993 the BJS estimated that there were 1.1 million cases of domestic abuse against women, a rate of 9.8 cases per 1,000 women. Five years later the rate had dropped to 7.5 cases per 1,000 women, a reduction of more than 25 percent. The rate of domestic abuse against males was largely unchanged over the same period. In 1993 the rate of domestic abuse against men was 1.6 per 1,000 males; in 1998 it was 1.5 per 1,000.

INJURY AND DEATH DUE TO ABUSE

The BJS found that most cases of domestic abuse involved simple assault, the use of force or the threat of force against another person. About 65 percent of domestic abuse against women and 68 percent of that against men consisted of simple assault. It is considered the least serious form of crime studied in the survey. Fifty percent of the female victims assaulted by partners suffered injuries, as compared to 32 percent of male victims. Most of those injuries were minor cuts or bruises. About 4 percent of injuries to female victims were serious; male victims sustained serious injuries in about 5 percent of cases. Only about 40 percent of victims, both male and female, sought medical treatment for their injuries. Most of those who did receive medical care received it at home or where the abuse occurred.

Unfortunately, many instances of domestic abuse end in the death of one or both partners. A 2001 BJS report titled *Intimate Partner Violence and Age of Victim* found that 1,218 women were murdered by current or former domestic partners in 1999. That represents more than three women killed each day by their partners. Domestic violence claimed 424 male homicide victims in 1999. According to the

Federal Bureau of Investigation's 1996 Uniform Crime Reports, current or former partners killed 30 percent of all female murder victims in the United States.

The rate of homicide among domestic partners has also been declining in recent years. Data from *Intimate Partner Violence* show that the number of women killed by intimate partners declined 23 percent between 1993 and 1997, although it increased by 8 percent between 1997 and 1998. Much of the decrease occurred among African-American females. The number of black females killed by their partners declined by 45 percent from 1976 to 1998. Murder rates for male victims also fell dramatically, dropping 44 percent for white males and 74 percent for black males. White females were the only group for whom the homicide rate among domestic partners has not decreased significantly. In fact, from 1997 to 1998, the number of white females killed by a partner rose 15 percent.

CHARACTERISTICS OF ABUSERS AND VICTIMS

No single "type" of person commits domestic abuse nor can a standard set of traits predict who will become an abuser. However, law enforcement agencies have studied both abusers and their victims and have come up with a list of characteristics common to many abusers. People who show these characteristics will not necessarily become abusers, but the presence of these factors may make them more likely to do so.

Intimate Partner Violence found that sex is the single most distinguishing characteristic of domestic abusers. Men commit most reported cases of domestic abuse and inflict much more damage than female abusers. Age was also closely linked to domestic violence. Women from ages 20 to 24 were most likely to be abused, with 21 cases of abuse per 1,000 women. Women under age 16 and over 50 suffered fewer than three victimizations per 1,000. By contrast, in no age group did the rate for males exceed three cases per 1,000.

Income and home ownership were also related to rates of domestic abuse. According to the BJS, lower-income households experienced significantly higher rates of domestic violence than those with higher incomes. The poorest women studied by the BJS suffered seven times more domestic violence than the wealthiest women. Renters also were much more likely to engage in domestic abuse than homeowners. Females in rental housing were three times more likely to be abused

DID YOU KNOW?

Murder of Intimate Partners, 1976–2000

| | Murder Victims of an Intimate Partner | | | |
| | Male | | Female | |
	Number	Percent of all murders	Number	Percent of all murders
1976	1,357	9.6%	1,600	34.9%
1980	1,221	6.9	1,549	29.6
1990	859	4.7	1,501	29.3
1993	708	3.7	1,581	28.5
2000	440	3.7	1,247	33.5

Source: Bureau of Justice Statistics, 2000.

than females who owned their own home. Male renters were more than twice as likely as male homeowners to be victims of domestic abuse. One theory of abuse suggests that those who live in poverty are under greater stress that those who do not have constant financial worries. These stresses can accumulate, causing frustration that may eventually lead to violence.

Race seems to be another factor influencing the rates of domestic violence. The BJS found that domestic violence occurred 35 percent more frequently to black females than to white females. Black men experienced 65 percent more domestic violence than white men. Black females and males both suffered domestic abuse at 22 times the rate of other, non-white races. There was no significant difference in the rate of domestic violence between Hispanic and non-Hispanic partners of either sex.

Where a person lives may also influence his or her chances of suffering from domestic violence. Urban women were much more likely than suburban women, and slightly more likely than rural women, to be victims of partner abuse. On the other hand, men in urban areas were no more likely than those in the suburbs to be abused by their partners. Urban males were only slightly more likely to be victims than rural dwellers. There was no significant difference between the rates of domestic violence among rural and suburban males.

REPORTING DOMESTIC ABUSE

The BJS estimates that only about half of all victims of domestic abuse report the crime to the police. Black women reported abuse far more often than any other group. In 1998, the BJS found that 67 percent of black women and 65 percent of Hispanic females who were abused filed a report with authorities, compared to 50 percent of white women, 48 percent of black men, and 45 percent of white men who were victims.

In an encouraging development, the percentage of victims who report abuse to the police has risen significantly since 1993. That year, according to the BJS, only about 48 percent of female abuse victims reported the incident to the police. In 1998 about 58 percent of female victims filed police reports. The rate of reporting by male victims has remained relatively unchanged over that period at about 50 percent.

Given the physical, emotional, and psychological damage caused by domestic abuse, why do so many victims never report abuse? In "Domestic Violence and the Criminal Justice System: An Overview," law professor Edna Erez examined research into the reasons for the underreporting of domestic abuse. These included:

- Shame or guilt about what victims see as their role in the abuse
- Fear of losing economic support from the abuser
- Concern for children and a desire to keep the family together
- Emotional attachment to the abuser
- Real or perceived lack of options if the victim leaves the abuser

According to *Intimate Partner Violence*, the reason given most often to the police for failure to report was that the abuse was "a private matter." This explanation was used by about half of all male victims and one-third of all female victims. About 19 percent of those who gave a reason for not reporting the abuse cited fear of reprisal. Around 10 percent said they didn't want to get their partner in trouble with the law.

Q & A

Question: My mother and stepfather fight a lot about me. I feel like it is my fault when he hits her. Is it my fault?

Answer: You are not at fault. Understand that your stepfather is not hitting your mom because of you. He is hitting her because he wants to control her. He would find other things to hit her for if you were not there. He probably tries to blame you, but he is responsible for his own actions. One of the traits of an abuser is to refuse to take responsibility and to blame everyone around him for "making him angry." Let your mother know you are scared and concerned about her safety and your own.

DOMESTIC PARTNER ABUSE IN SAME-SEX RELATIONSHIPS

Domestic partner abuse is not limited to heterosexual couples. A 1997 report by the National Coalition of Anti-Violence Programs (NCAVP) was one of the first to explore violence in same-sex relationships in depth. Prior to the study, titled "The Prevalence of Lesbian, Gay, Bisexual, and Transgender Domestic Violence," fewer than a dozen scholarly studies had been conducted on the topic of violence in same-sex relationships.

The NCAVP report found that 3,327 cases of domestic abuse were reported among lesbian, gay, bisexual, and transgender couples in 1997. This represented an increase of 41 percent over the number of cases reported the previous year. Male victims reported 52 percent of those cases of abuse, while females reported 48 percent. The NCAVP suggests that only a fraction of the number of actual assaults is ever reported to the police.

Same-sex victims, like heterosexual victims, may be reluctant to seek help from the police, courts, or social services. Many fear they will experience prejudice because of their sexual orientation, and there is some evidence that those fears are justified. Some same-sex partners report that the police do not take the incident as seriously as they would a man beating his wife. Some gay victims claim that police occasionally make antigay comments or even engage in antigay violence.

Same-sex victims often have difficulty obtaining the social services available to battered women. Some 25 agencies that belong to the

NCAVP offer help to victims of hate crimes such as antigay violence, but less than half help victims of domestic abuse. Most shelters and programs are set up to help heterosexual women fleeing their abusive boyfriends or husbands. They are not set up for men—gay or straight. Staff members at most clinics or social services agencies are often less knowledgeable about and less compassionate toward, same-sex victims of domestic abuse.

RESPONDING TO DOMESTIC ABUSE

The NCADV stresses that anyone living with an abuser should plan for his or her safety. He or she should:

- Have a safe place to go during an argument
- Think about people to contact who can provide a safe place to stay
- Carry change for a phone call at all times
- Establish a "code word" or sign to give to friends and family so they can call for help
- Plan what to say to a partner if he or she becomes violent
- Remember that everyone has the right to live without fear and violence

The NCADV also suggests safety planning for victims who have left the relationship. Steps a person can take to protect himself or herself against continuing abuse from a former partner include:

- Changing one's phone number
- Screening phone calls
- Documenting all contacts, messages, and injuries involving the batterer
- Changing the locks on all doors
- Planning how to get away if confronted by an abusive partner
- Meeting only in public places with a former partner
- Varying daily routines
- Calling a shelter for advice and information
- Keeping important documents on hand so one can apply for legal or financial help

All states now have laws against domestic abuse. These laws state that threatening or striking a partner is a crime. The severity of the crime depends on such factors as the use of weapons, injuries, and age of the victim. Many states also now have mandatory arrest laws that require police officers to arrest an abuser if they have good reason to believe an assault has occurred.

If the attacker is arrested, he or she is jailed and then appears before a judge. However, the attacker often is released on bail and the victim remains in danger. In such cases a **restraining order** can help. A restraining order is a document that orders the abuser to stay away from his or her victim. Violations of the provisions of the order may result in jail time. The abuser may also be ordered to attend a treatment program. An order of protection may also grant the victim custody of the children, financial support, and possession of the house or car. In some cases, if the abuser even tries to call his or her victim, he or she can be arrested.

An order of protection can give the victim some legal protection, but it does not provide for his or her physical safety. Leaving an abusive relationship can be dangerous and the order of protection may incite the abuser to further violence. It is important for the victim (and any children) to have a safe place or shelter that the abuser can't reach by phone or in person. Getting the victim away from the abuse is the first step in a longer process that will enable her to live independently, restore self-esteem, and enter into healthier relationships.

See also: Abuse in Society; Abuse, Theories of; Abuse, Witnesses of; Abusers, Common Traits of; Legal Intervention; Men and Abuse; Rehabilitation and Treatment; Stalking; Women and Abuse

FURTHER READING

Bancroft, Lundy, and Jay G. Silverman. *The Batterer as Parent: Addressing the Impact of Domestic Violence on Family Dynamics.* Thousand Oaks, CA: Sage Publications, 2002.

Schlesinger Buzawa, Eva, and Carl G. Buzawa. *Domestic Violence: The Criminal Justice Response, Third Edition.* Thousand Oaks, CA: Sage Publications, 2002.

Davis, Richard L. *Domestic Violence: Facts and Fallacies.* New York: Praeger Publishers, 1998.

Hamberger, L. Kevin, and Claire Renzetti. 1996. *Domestic Partner Abuse.* New York: Springer Publishing Company.

Harway, Michele. What Causes Men's Violence against Women? Thousand Oaks, CA: Sage Publications, 1999.

■ ELDER ABUSE

The use of physical, emotional, or verbal violence to control a dependent elderly person. Senior citizens are particularly vulnerable to abuse because they are more likely to suffer from physical or mental impairments that make them dependent on others for basic physical, medical, emotional, or financial needs. Like other forms of abuse, most elder abuse is committed by relatives or other **caregivers**. Elder abuse also resembles other forms of abuse in that many cases go unreported.

TYPES OF ELDER ABUSE

There are several forms of elder abuse. According to the National Center on Elder Abuse (NCEA), these types of abuse include:

- **Physical abuse**, which includes hitting, shoving, kicking, burning, shaking, pushing, grabbing or handling roughly. It also includes the use of physical restraint, force-feeding, or inappropriately forcing an elderly person to take drugs.

- **Emotional abuse**, which involves inflicting pain or distress through verbal or nonverbal acts. Verbal acts include name-calling, insults, threats, and harassment. Nonverbal acts include forced social isolation or treating an elderly person as if he or she were incompetent.

- Financial exploitation, which involves taking improper control over the victim's money, property, or other assets. The caregiver or relative may be guilty of theft, fraud, or misuse of the older person's money. Financial exploitation also involves forging the signature of an elderly person in one's care or deceiving him or her into signing a legal document such as a will. (Institutions such as nursing homes commit financial abuse when they charge for services that are not provided or requested.)

- Sexual abuse, sexual assault, and sexual harassment, which affect older people as well as those who are young. The abuse includes, but is not limited to, unwanted touching, forced nudity, sexually explicit photographing, and all types of sexual assault or battery including rape.

■ Neglect, which is the failure to provide for the basic medical or practical needs of the older person. Examples of neglect include failing to provide adequate food, shelter, grooming, clothes, or access to a bathroom. Abandonment occurs when a caregiver leaves a dependent senior alone in the home or fails to show up to provide care.

■ Self-neglect, which is behavior by a mentally competent elderly person that threatens his or her own welfare. It includes refusing adequate food, water, clothing, shelter, hygiene, medication, or safety.

Q & A

Question: What are the signs that elder abuse may be occurring?

Answer: The NCEA lists a number of signs that an elderly person may be the victim of abuse. Signs of physical abuse include:

■ Bruises, black eyes, welts, or rope marks

■ Sprains, dislocations, fractures, or internal injuries

■ Open wounds or cuts, or untreated injuries

■ Sudden changes in the elderly person's behavior

■ The caregiver refuses to let visitors see the elder in private

Signs of emotional or psychological abuse include the following:

■ Distress or agitation

■ Withdrawal or refusal to communicate

■ Unusual behavior such as sucking, rocking, or biting

Signs of financial exploitation include the following:

■ Sudden changes in banking or spending habits

■ Disappearance of money or possessions

■ Sudden transfers of money to a relative or other person

■ Sudden changes to wills or financial documents

■ The addition of names to an elder's bank card

■ Poor level of care for the elder despite adequate finances to provide proper care

Signs of neglect include the following:

■ Dehydration, malnutrition, poor hygiene, bed sores

■ Untreated health problems

■ Unsafe housing or living conditions, for example a lack of heat or running water

■ Unsanitary or unclean living conditions

In addition to the signals listed above, any report of abuse by an elderly person should be taken seriously.

RATES OF ELDER ABUSE

According to the NCEA, elder abuse is greatly underreported. In its 1996 report "Trends in Elder Abuse in Domestic Settings," the NCEA cites statistics that estimate only one in every 14 incidents of elder abuse that occur in the home are reported. A May 2002 article for the NCEA newsletter titled "Abuse in Nursing Homes" found that abuse in institutional settings such as nursing homes is also significantly underreported.

The numbers that are available suggest a widespread problem, especially considering how few cases of elder abuse are reported. In the NCEA's 2000 State Adult Protective Services Survey, state agencies reported 472,813 cases of elder abuse. Family members filed most complaints of elder abuse (13.7 percent of the total). Health care workers such as private physicians and nursing home employees reported 11.1 percent of the cases, social service agencies reported 10 percent, and law enforcement officers reported 9.5 percent. Only 8 percent of all cases were reported by the victim.

The NCEA report found that Caucasians and women over the age of 60 were the groups most likely to be victims of elder abuse. Women represented 56 percent of all cases of elder abuse in the United States in 2000. Some 39 percent of cases involved men; in the remaining cases the victim's sex was not specified. Almost two-thirds (65.8 percent) of the cases of elder abuse involved Caucasians, while 17.4 percent involved African Americans and 10.5 percent involved Latinos. Native Americans, Asians, and Pacific Islanders each represented less than 1 percent of all reported elder abuse cases.

A troubling finding in the NCEA report is that the rate of abuse appears to increase with age. Adults in the oldest category surveyed by the NCEA—80 years and older—were victims in 46.5 percent of cases of elder abuse. This same age group also accounted for more cases of self-neglect than any other group—33.6 percent.

WHO ABUSES THE ELDERLY?

Rates of elder abuse are less likely to vary by gender than the rates for child abuse. In 1996 the NCEA found that women committed 48.9 percent of all cases of elder abuse in the United States in 1996, while men committed 47.4 percent. In the remaining 3.7 percent, the sex of the perpetrator was unknown or unreported. According to the 2000 State Adult Protective Services Survey, 52 percent of the identified perpetrators of elder abuse were men.

Most of the perpetrators in the 2000 State Adult Protective Services Survey (24.8 percent) were between the ages of 36 and 50. Those between the ages of 18 and 35 made up 18.5 percent of all offenders, while individuals under 18 accounted for only 5.9 percent of all perpetrators. However, in almost one-third of the reported cases (31.6 percent), the offender's age was not given.

Some professionals say that elder abuse is "domestic violence grown old," meaning that spouses who abused their partners in younger years continue to abuse them in old age. Statistics from the NCEA report tend to bear out this argument. Spouses or intimate partners commit over 30 percent of all cases of elder abuse. Adult children account for 17.6 percent of cases, and family members as a whole were involved in 61.7 percent of elder abuse cases. In 11.3 percent of the cases the abuser was listed as unknown, and in 10.5 percent of cases the relationship of the perpetrator of the abuse was classified as "other."

The NCEA report found that staff at nursing homes and other institutions caring for the elderly committed only 4.4 percent of all reported elder abuse. However, a 1990 article in the *Journal of Elder Abuse and Neglect* showed that abuse in institutional settings is widespread. The article "Highlights from a Study of Abuse of Patients in Nursing Homes" reported the results of interviews with 577 nurses and nurses' aides working with the elderly. Some 10 percent of the nurses and aides admitted to physically abusing residents at least once in the previous year. Forty percent had psychologically abused residents in the past year. Over a third (36 percent) said they had seen another staff member physically abuse a resident, and 81 percent had observed psychological abuse.

Fact Or Fiction?

Nursing homes are the safest places for elderly people with physical or mental problems.

Fact: Although some nursing homes are safe, many are guilty of neglecting and abusing the seniors in their care. A study commissioned by U.S. Representative Henry Waxman of California found that 5,283 of the approximately 17,000 nursing homes in the United States had been cited for abuse in 1999 and 2000. More than 1,600 of the homes committed violations that could place residents in immediate danger of serious injury or death. In 256 homes, abuse violations actually resulted in death or serious injury.

The report cited instances of "appalling physical, sexual, and verbal abuse." These included an incident where a nursing home worker struck a resident in the face and broke her nose. In another case, a male nurse attempted to rape a resident in her room. Unfortunately, the problem seems to be growing. According to the study, twice as many nursing homes were cited for abuse in 2000 as in 1996.

RISK FACTORS FOR ELDER ABUSE

Several theories have been proposed to explain the causes of elder abuse, but few have been thoroughly tested. The NCEA, however, has identified several factors that may increase the risk that person will become an elder abuser.

- Substance abuse. According to the National Committee for the Prevention of Elder Abuse, drug and alcohol abuse is the most often cited risk factor for elder abuse. Substance abusers may see elderly relatives as a source of money for their drug habit or may use their homes as a base for drug dealing. Elderly spouses who abuse their partners are more likely to be violent under the influence of alcohol or drugs.

- Continuing partner abuse. The NCEA reports that a large percentage of cases of elder abuse involves couples with a history of domestic partner abuse. If one spouse or partner has historically tried to control the actions of the other, that behavior may well continue into old age.

- Personal problems. In many cases of elder abuse, the abuser is a caregiver who is financially dependent upon an elderly relative because of personal problems such as substance abuse or mental health problems. Adult children with such problems seem to be particularly likely to abuse elderly parents in their care.

- Social isolation. Those who abuse elders may be more likely to be isolated (or to isolate themselves) from social contact with other people besides the victim.

- Caregiver stress. A popular theory states that caregivers become overwhelmed by the task of caring for elderly relatives and may react by harming the elderly person in some way. Few cases of abuse that have been studied closely, however, fit this pattern.

- Characteristics of the victim. Some theories suggest that certain traits of the victim—such as dementia (a loss of mental and emotional functioning often associated with aging), personality disorders, or disruptive behavior— may increase his or her risk of suffering abuse.

GETTING HELP

Help is available for elder abuse—if it is reported. Relatives need to stay involved and monitor the health of the elderly person. They also need to make sure he or she is not socially isolated and that one family member does not have sole responsibility for financial or medical decisions (unless the senior has made that decision on his or her own.) If abuse by a relative is suspected, friends or other relatives may need to get involved to prevent further injury. A concerned relative or friend can also report suspected abuse to the authorities and an investigation will begin. The report can be anonymous.

In most states, an adult protective services agency is the primary agency responsible for investigating reports of elder abuse. This agency is often part of the social services department in a city or county. If the agency finds that abuse or neglect has occurred, it makes arrangements to care for and protect the victim. Other agencies or institutions that are also involved in helping vulnerable seniors include state social service departments, law enforcement agencies, hospitals and medical facilities, and mental health departments. The federal law known as the 1975 Older Americans Act also created a long-term care ombudsman (official investigator) to check out complaints about mistreatment or poor conditions in nursing homes.

If there is any suspicion of elder abuse by a paid caregiver, a relative should report it to the agency that placed the worker and then ask for another employee. The relative can also change agencies and report the abuse to the authorities. If the elder is in immediate danger, the police should be called right away. The keys to combating elder abuse are keeping a close eye on the well-being of elderly people in the care of others and acting quickly if you suspect abuse may be occurring.

See also: Alcohol, Drugs, and Abuse; Domestic Partner Abuse; Legal Intervention

FURTHER READING

Bennett, Gary. *Elder Abuse: Concepts, Theories, and Interventions.* London: Chapman and Hall, 1994.

Brownell, Patricia J. *Family Crimes against the Elderly: Elder Abuse and the Criminal Justice System.* Hamden, CT: Garland Publishing, 1998.

Hird, Mary. *Elder Abuse, Neglect, and Maltreatment: What Can Be Done to Stop It.* Pittsburgh, PA: Dorrance Publishing Company, 2003.

Quinn, Mary Joy, and Susan K. Tomita. *Elder Abuse and Neglect: Causes, Diagnosis, and Intervention Strategies.* New York: Springer Publishing Company, 1997.

■ HARASSMENT

See: Bullying; Elder Abuse; Sexual Abuse; Women and Abuse

■ HAZING

Playing humiliating pranks or practical jokes on an individual as a form of initiation into a group, club, or society. Hazing is a widespread practice in high schools and colleges, especially among sports teams, **peer** groups, and student organizations such as music or theater clubs. Initiation rites typically involve harmless activities such as dressing in embarrassing costumes. However, in some cases hazing can include dangerous acts such as **physical abuse** or forced consumption of large quantities of alcohol.

Clearly, hazing activities that threaten the health or well-being of an individual are harmful and unacceptable. However, even acts that seem relatively harmless, such as being forced to publicly embarrass oneself, can cause psychological harm to the victim. In recent years, the public has been increasingly concerned about the rise in the number of violent and even fatal hazing incidents. Controlling the types of behavior that take place at initiation ceremonies and eliminating dangerous hazing practices have become a significant challenge for school officials and anti-hazing organizations.

WHAT CONSTITUTES HAZING?

Not all initiation rites are considered hazing. In fact, according to a major study on hazing conducted by Alfred University, initiation into a group can serve as a positive social experience. However, it is important to distinguish between what constitutes positive initiation ceremonies and hazing.

Constructive initiation rites

Learning how to get along with others and gain social acceptance from one's peers is one of the developmental challenges of adolescence. Alfred University's 1999 study, "Initiation Rites in American High Schools: A National Survey" states that properly conducted initiation ceremonies can help teens better meet that challenge. The study claims that initiation can serve important social goals, including:

- meeting teens' need for a sense of belonging
- helping members understand the history and culture of the group; and
- building relationships with others in the group.

The Alfred University study defines positive initiation rites as "pro-social behaviors that build social relationships, understanding, empathy, civility, altruism, and moral decision making." The study found that 98 percent of the teens it surveyed took part in at least one such "community-building initiation activity." These activities include:

- Maintaining a specific grade point average (GPA)
- Tryouts, auditions, or other relevant tests of skill
- Going on field trips, challenge courses, or practice events
- Participating in group projects, fund-raisers, or work camps
- Dressing up formally for club events
- Playing games or sports as a group
- Taking oaths or signing contracts
- Mentoring, tutoring, or being a Big Brother/Big Sister

According to the survey, females and students with high GPAs were the groups most likely to participate in community-building initiation activities rather than hazing. Teens who did not know an adult who experienced hazing were more likely to take part in constructive initiation activities. So were teens who did not know adults who considered hazing socially acceptable.

In fact, when most teens think of initiation, they think of these positive activities rather than hazing. When asked to name the kinds of activities that would be expected of them when they joined a group, most teens in the Alfred University survey mentioned positive activities. Three times as many teens named activities such as community service or being role models than those who mentioned humiliating or dangerous hazing activities.

Fact Or Fiction?

Hazing involves foolish pranks. No harm is done.

Fact: Hazing is about power and control over others. Even if injury is not intended, the degradation and humiliation is intentional. Serious accidents do occur, even during "innocent" activities such as scavenger hunts. The hazing does not establish order or respect for leaders of sports teams, fraternities, or other groups. Leadership is established by mutual respect, and respect must be earned; it cannot be imposed by force. Hazing breeds disrespect, mistrust, and even fear.

Destructive initiation rites

While constructive initiation rites can be a strong source of positive socialization, hazing has no such redeeming qualities. The Alfred

University study defined hazing as "any humiliating or dangerous activity expected of you to join in a group, regardless of your willingness to participate." The survey divided hazing activities into three broad categories: humiliation, substance abuse, and dangerous hazing.

Humiliation consisted of such behaviors as being yelled, cursed, or sworn at; being forced to associate with certain people and avoid others; acting as a servant to older group members; being forced to undress in public; being required to tell dirty jokes or stories; and other forms of public embarrassment. Some hazing requires that participants get tattooed, pierce parts of their body, or shave off all of their hair. Humiliation may also involve eating or drinking disgusting things and depriving oneself of food, sleep, or hygiene.

Substance abuse includes drinking alcohol, taking part in drinking contests, drinking until one loses consciousness, smoking huge quantities of cigarettes or cigars, or using illegal drugs. Dangerous hazing may include acts such as harassing other people, vandalizing property, stealing or committing some other crime, getting into fights, inflicting pain on oneself, allowing oneself to be tied up or exposed to extreme cold, being beaten or physically abused, and being cruel to animals.

The Alfred University study found that humiliation is a strong warning that illegal hazing activities are occurring or are likely to occur. Over half (56 percent) of the teens surveyed were not only humiliated as part of initiation ceremonies but also forced to engage in dangerous and potentially illegal acts. This finding refutes the claim by many advocates of hazing that such activities are merely youthful pranks and not something that needs to be taken seriously.

INCIDENCE OF HAZING

Although the majority of high school students associate initiation with positive activities, a significant number of teens are victims of hazing. Forty-eight percent of the teens surveyed by Alfred University reported being subjected to some kind of hazing. Based on the figures from the study, about 1.5 million high school students in the United States suffer some form of hazing every year.

Almost all of the hazing victims in the study (and about 43 percent of all students surveyed) had been subjected to humiliation. In addition, 23 percent of students were asked to participate in substance abuse as part of their initiations. About 29 percent of the students surveyed were expected to take part in some kind of illegal activity, including substance abuse. Twenty-two percent of students experienced dangerous hazing, such as physical abuse or participating in violence or serious criminal activity.

The groups most likely to subject members to hazing are fraternities and sororities, gangs, and other peer groups. Only 6 percent of all college students belong to fraternities or sororities, but 76 percent of those who do are subjected to hazing. Peer groups and gangs haze about 73 percent of their members. Sixty-seven percent of the teens in the survey participated in sports, and 35 percent of teens on sports teams had been hazed. Almost a quarter of all the teens (24 percent) in the Alfred University study reported being hazed as part of a sports team.

Surprisingly, even groups generally associated with positive values and activities are prone to hazing. Among students who joined vocational groups such as cheerleading squads or bands, 27 percent reported being hazed. Church groups, which include 29 percent of all high school students, subjected 24 percent of their members to hazing. Other organizations where hazing is frequent include political and social action groups; music, theater, and art clubs; and social organizations. Scholastic clubs were much less likely than other groups to engage in hazing. However, the study found that, when they do haze, they tend to engage in dangerous activities.

VICTIMS OF HAZING

According to the Alfred University study, no group in high school is completely free from hazing. However, certain groups are more likely to experience hazing or to haze others. Students' attitudes toward hazing can be significantly affected by adult influences in their lives. In the study, students who knew an adult who was hazed were more likely to be hazed than those who did not. A student is also more likely to haze others if adults in the student's life consider hazing socially acceptable. Students who consider hazing socially acceptable are more likely both to participate in and to suffer from hazing.

Boys are more likely than girls to take part in hazing and are significantly more likely to engage in dangerous hazing activities. Among the boys surveyed by Alfred University, 48 percent suffered humiliation hazing, 27 percent took part in dangerous hazing, and 24 percent engaged in substance abuse. By comparison, 39 percent of girls reported humiliation hazing, 18 percent were involved in substance abuse, and 17 percent underwent dangerous hazing.

In many cases, hazing was found to start much earlier than high school. One out of every four students who reported being hazed in high school said they were hazed before they were teenagers. Ten percent of the students surveyed by Alfred University were nine years old or younger when they were first hazed. Another 15 percent first experienced hazing between the ages of 10 and 12. The majority of students (61 percent) underwent hazing for the first time between ages 13 and 15.

The type of hazing students experience also varies by the type of groups they join. For example, members of cheerleading and other vocational groups were likely to suffer humiliation and substance abuse but unlikely to engage in dangerous hazing. Political groups were also likely to include substance abuse in their hazing activities. By contrast, scholastic groups were less likely to humiliate their members or subject them to substance abuse. However, they were significantly high in the incidence of dangerous hazing. Sports teams, gangs, peer groups, fraternities, sororities, and music/art/theater groups rated high in all forms of hazing. Surprisingly, nearly half of the students hazed by church groups were expected to engage in illegal activities.

TEENS SPEAK

I Finally Found Out What the Big Secret Was

I was really excited to join the basketball team this year, especially because I had just missed making it last year. After one of my friends, Sean, made the team last year he told me he had to go through an initiation before he was accepted as part of the team. I asked him what he had to do, but he wouldn't say. He told me it was secret and that if I wanted to find out I had to make the team. Well, now I know why it was a secret.

When the final list of team members was announced on Friday, the captain told us to meet in the gym after school. At the meeting, the new members (me and two other guys named Darrell and Mike) were told to strip down to our shorts. The other team members then took our clothes and told us we had to get home wearing nothing but our underwear. That was bad enough, but it was really cold outside and it looked like it might snow. The captain just joked that we'd stay warm if we moved fast enough, "and you'll be moving fast, believe me!"

By the time the other guys left, it was starting to get dark, so Darrell, Mike, and I decided to wait a few minutes and then go. We wanted to make sure none of the guys was waiting to soak us with a hose or something like that. Luckily there was no one in the school parking lot when we ran across it. We then split up and each headed for home. I was dodging between hedges and houses to keep out of sight, but sometimes I had to run out in the open. A lot of people saw me and laughed. After about 20 minutes it started snowing and then I was really miserable.

By the time I got home I was frozen to the bone. My mom hit the roof when she saw me and told me to take a bath and get into bed. I was sick for the next three days. My dad really chewed me out for pulling such a stupid stunt, but he seemed to mellow out a little when I told him it was a team initiation. He said he went through something like that when he joined the football team at school. Still, he wasn't happy about what I did, and he grounded me for a week. The next time I hear about a "cool" secret initiation, I'll think twice about wanting to join that group.

CONSEQUENCES OF HAZING

An incident in 2003 offers an extreme example of what can happen when hazing gets out of hand. Five high school junior girls went to the hospital after a hazing incident in suburban Chicago. It started as a traditional touch football game between senior and junior girls to initiate the latter into the senior class. Juniors expected some humiliation such as having ketchup or mustard smeared in their hair, but what they got was completely unexpected. One girl reported being strangled and kicked repeatedly in the head. Some of the senior girls brought baseball bats to strike the juniors. Bystanders—including some male students—were even allowed to participate.

Although what happened in Chicago was clearly not the norm, all forms of hazing can result in a wide range of emotional, psychological, medical, and legal problems. Almost three quarters (71 percent) of the high school students studied by Alfred University reported suffering one or more negative consequences of hazing. The types of negative consequences they mentioned (and the percentage of students who suffered from each consequence) include:

- Getting into a fight (24 percent)
- Suffering an injury (23 percent)
- Fighting with parents (22 percent)
- Poor school performance (21 percent)
- Injuring another person (20 percent)
- Missing school, sports practice, a game, or a meeting (19 percent)
- Difficulty eating, sleeping, or concentrating (18 percent)
- Committing a crime (16 percent)
- Suicidal thoughts (15 percent)
- Getting sick (12 percent)
- No longer going out with friends (11 percent)
- Getting in trouble with the police (10 percent)
- Convicted of a crime (4 percent)

Other negative consequences reported by students included **depression,** fighting with family members other than parents, feeling tormented or made fun of at school, low self-esteem, suffering insults, and having an emotional breakdown.

Students expressed a mixture of emotions when asked to express their feelings about being hazed. Twenty-seven percent of the students who had been hazed said they had negative feelings about the experience, 27 percent had positive feelings, and 32 percent had both positive and negative feelings. For 14 percent, the only feeling they felt was a desire for revenge against those who hazed them.

Negative feelings reported by the students included anger, embarrassment, confusion, guilt, regret, sadness, betrayal, loneliness, worthlessness, self-hatred, and feelings of being stupid and dirty. Among the positive feelings mentioned were group identity, pride, strength, excitement, happiness, confidence, self-esteem, and a sense of being trusted or part of a family. Many of the students (29 percent) were simply relieved the ordeal was over or glad to know that others had gone through it as well.

CONFRONTING AND PREVENTING HAZING

The researchers at Alfred University not only asked high school students about their experiences with hazing but also what students felt were the best ways to stop hazing. Twenty-seven percent of students said that hazing is an ingrained part of American culture and felt that only drastic changes in the culture could prevent it. Students agreed that it was up to parents and other role models to teach children proper behavior from an early age, including speaking out against hazing. Adults also need to reward students for reporting or publicly condemning hazing. The students also felt that it was the responsibility of teens themselves to pressure their peers not to engage in hazing.

The majority of students (61 percent) called for strict rules against hazing with strong enforcement of the rules. Half said that the police should investigate and prosecute hazing as a way to discourage it. They mentioned strategies such as zero-tolerance policies, disbanding any group that engages in hazing, expelling students who haze, and sentencing perpetrators to jail time.

Other recommended strategies included more activities designed to provide alternatives to hazing. Students suggested such things as mentally challenging activities, spiritual or church involvement, and extracurricular programs for teens. Some suggested holding classes to educate students about the dangers of hazing. Others felt that schools should inform parents about any initiation rites that take place at school or club activities. Parents should know the school's policy on hazing and be asked to help prevent hazing. These suggestions reflect the larger idea that parents and other adults close to teens should become more aware of hazing.

Q & A

Question: What steps can be taken to prevent hazing?

Answer: The Alfred University hazing study included the following recommendations for preventing hazing.

■ Educate school leaders, community leaders, parents, and students on hazing and its consequences.

■ Include student behavior as part of school leaders' performance evaluations.

■ Have students and parents sign an anti-hazing contract.

■ Require certain standards of academic performance and behavior to participate in extracurricular activities.

■ Take strong disciplinary action against hazing, including notifying law enforcement authorities.

104 The Truth About Abuse

- Place greater value on community, equality, and civility.
- Train adult and student leaders in community-building initiation activities and reward them for successful efforts.
- Provide opportunities for supervised play for younger children and community service experiences for teens.
- Teach children right from wrong and train them to be conscious of the feelings of others.
- Encourage kids not to keep secrets, especially about hazing or other abuse.
- Give kids a way to report hazing without having to go public.
- Pay particular attention to students who are excluded from group activities or who express a desire for revenge.

At the heart of the Alfred University recommendations are three basic ideas:

1. Authority figures need to send a clear anti-hazing message to students.
2. The larger culture must change to place greater value on the community.
3. Parents, teachers, and peers need to pay attention to kids who are socially isolated.

Putting these ideas into practice requires the efforts of parents, educators, and community leaders, as well as teens themselves—a community working as a team to fight hazing.

See also: Alcohol, Drugs, and Abuse

FURTHER READING
Nuwer, Hank. *The Hazing Reader.* Bloomington: Indiana University Press, 2004.
Nuwer, Hank. *Wrongs of Passage: Fraternities, Sororities, Hazing, and Binge Drinking.* Bloomington: Indiana University Press, 2002.
Schleifer, Joe. 1996. *Everything You Need to Know about the Dangers of Hazing.* New York: Rosen Publishing Group, 1996.

■ HOMICIDE

The deliberate taking of another person's life. Abuse can have many tragic consequences, but clearly the most extreme of these is homicide, or murder. Each year, thousands of Americans of all ages and both sexes are victims of homicide. Most of these cases involve the murder of a spouse or intimate partner, although each year hundreds of parents also murder their own children.

DOMESTIC PARTNER HOMICIDE

The Federal Bureau of Investigation (FBI) and the Department of Justice (DOJ) compile extensive statistics annually on all forms of violent crime, including murder. According to the FBI, 14,054 murders occurred in the United States in 2002, a rate of 5.6 murders per 100,000 people. The rate shows a decline over the previous year, thus continuing a trend that began in the early 1990s of steadily declining murder rates. In 10,779 of those cases, the victims were males. Female murder victims in 2002 numbered 3,251.

Although significantly more men than women are victims of homicide every year, domestic violence claims more female victims and accounts for a much larger proportion of the women who are murdered. Men are much more likely than women to be killed by a stranger or during the course of another crime such as robbery. Women are far more likely to be killed by a spouse or other domestic partner. Wives or girlfriends killed 287 of the nearly 11,000 men murdered in 2002 (2.7 percent of all murders involving male victims). By contrast, boyfriends or husbands killed 1,045 of the 3,251 female murder victims (32 percent of all homicides in female victims).

As with homicide rates in general, the rate of homicide among domestic partners has been declining in recent years. Data from the DOJ report *Intimate Partner Violence* show that the number of women killed by intimate partners declined 23 percent between 1993 and 1997. The greatest decline was among male victims of domestic violence. The murder rate fell 44 percent for white male victims and 74 percent for black male victims during this period. By contrast, the murder rate among white female domestic partners rose 15 percent over the same period.

HOMICIDE RELATED TO CHILD ABUSE

In 2002, a total of 1,357 children in the United States under the age of 18 were murder victims. As with adult victims of abuse, male children suffered more total homicides, while female children were more likely to be killed by a loved one. Males accounted for 867 of the victims, with 239 of those victims (27.6 percent) being killed by their parents. There were 489 female children murdered in 2002; of those 210, 42.9 percent were murdered by their parents.

Some observers claim that official government statistics on child murder underestimate the extent of the problem. A 1999 report by the Department of Health and Human Services that reviewed 10 years of death records from North Carolina found that state record keepers had failed to list abuse or battering as the cause of death in 58.7 percent of the child homicide cases over that period of time. The report estimated that the number of deaths due to child abuse is probably underestimated by 61.6 percent. If the estimate was accurate, the number of children murdered by their parents in 2002 would rise from the official total of 499 to 1,154.

Other organizations argue that even these figures severely underestimate the extent of the problem. The U.S. Advisory Board on Child Abuse and Neglect calculates that about 2,000 children a year die as a result or abuse or neglect. Researchers believe the number is underreported because many deaths are misidentified as Sudden Infant Death Syndrome or as accidents.

HOMICIDE LAWS

The intentions of the killer define two broad categories of murder: murder in the first degree and murder in the second degree. In first-degree murder, the perpetrator plans to kill his or her victim before committing the crime. This kind of homicide is also called premeditated (thought out beforehand) murder. Second-degree murder occurs when a perpetrator kills a victim during an emotional or violent episode—in "the heat of the moment." For example, if a husband becomes enraged while arguing with his wife and beats her so badly that she dies from the injuries, he is likely to be charged with second-degree murder.

Both forms of murder are felonies, serious crimes punishable by a sentence in a state or federal prison. The punishment for murder varies from state to state, and the federal government has its own guidelines that differ from those of the states. In most states, second-degree murder is punishable by a prison term that can range from 10 years to life. Ten years is also the minimum punishment for first-degree murder in most states. The maximum punishment for homicide in most states is death. However, 13 states have outlawed the death penalty. In those

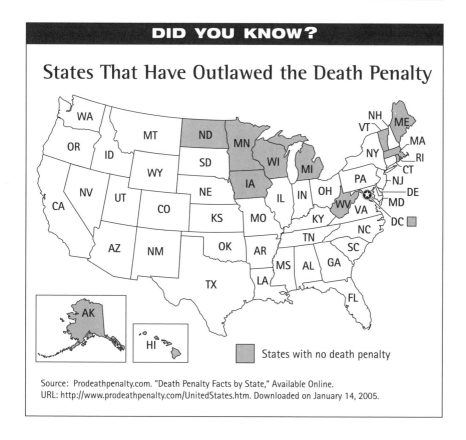

DID YOU KNOW?

States That Have Outlawed the Death Penalty

States with no death penalty

Source: Prodeathpenalty.com. "Death Penalty Facts by State," Available Online.
URL: http://www.prodeathpenalty.com/UnitedStates.htm. Downloaded on January 14, 2005.

states, the maximum punishment for murder is life in prison without the possibility of **parole**, or early release from prison.

MOTIVATIONS AND RESPONSES

Most cases of murder involving domestic partners are considered second-degree murder. According to the FBI's Uniform Crime Reports, most murders of domestic partners (58 percent) occur as the result of an argument. The causes of over a third of such murders (37 percent) are classified as "other" or "unknown." Clearly, much of the deadly violence that occurs between domestic partners happens when one or both parties are unable to maintain emotional control in a tense situation. In situations where one partner is physically much stronger than the other, or in which one partner has access to a weapon, the potential for deadly violence is much greater.

In many cases, women who kill their partners do so in self-defense. A 1986 article from the journal *Law and Contemporary Problems* titled "Husband-Wife Homicide: An Essay from a Family Law Perspective" reported the results of a University of Florida research study. Researchers found that most of the women who had killed their husbands had endured "prolonged physical or verbal abuse." They also learned that lethal violence is particularly likely when a wife tries to leave an abusive relationship. According to the study, abusive husbands are often killed while trying to physically prevent their wives from leaving.

Fact Or Fiction?

Men who kill their domestic partners receive longer prison sentences than women convicted of the same crime.

Fact: According to the Department of Justice report "Violence against Intimates," the average prison sentence for men who kill their wives is 17.5 years. The average sentence for women who kill their husbands is 6.2 years. Differences in sentencing often reflect circumstances surrounding the case, such as a wife's claims of self-defense or a history of abusive or violent behavior by the husband.

The National Coalition Against Domestic Violence (NCADV) urges anyone living with an abuser to plan for his or her own safety. Whenever the potential for deadly domestic violence exists, such a plan can be a lifesaver. According to the NCADV, a person who fears that a spouse or partner may be capable of lethal violence should:

- Have a safe place to go during an argument
- Contact relatives or friends who can provide a safe place to stay
- Carry a cell phone or change for a phone call at all times
- Establish a "code word" or sign to give to friends and family so they can call for help
- Decide what to say to a partner if he or she becomes violent

Since domestic violence is particularly likely when a victim leaves an abusive relationship, the NCADV also suggests that those who have left make a safety plan as well. Steps that can increase one's safety include:

- Changing one's phone number
- Screening phone calls
- Changing the locks on all doors
- Planning how to get away if confronted by the former partner
- Meeting only in public places with a former partner
- Varying daily routines

Although only a small percentage of all abusive relationships end in homicide, the potential for violence is often present. People who would never consciously consider murdering a partner may—and often do—kill, either in a fit of rage or in self-defense. Knowing how to avoid, defuse, or escape a potentially violent confrontation can mean the difference between life and death.

See also: Child Abuse; Domestic Partner Abuse; Women and Abuse

FURTHER READING
Browne, Angela. *When Battered Women Kill.* New York: Free Press, 1989.
Moffatt, Gregory K. *Blindsided: Homicide Where You Least Expect It.* New York: Praeger Publishers, 2000.
Women's Coalition Against Family Violence. *Blood on Whose Hands? The Killing of Women and Children in Domestic Homicides.* Annandale, AU: The Federation Press, 1994.

■ LEGAL INTERVENTION
Actions taken by police or the courts to prevent abuse, prosecute and punish perpetrators of abuse, and protect victims from further abuse. **Physical abuse**, sexual abuse, and **neglect** are illegal in all 50 states. Some states also have laws that prohibit emotional, psychological, and financial abuse. Specific laws vary from state to state.

DOMESTIC PARTNER ABUSE LAWS
Both state and federal law offer protection to victims of domestic partner abuse. The Violence Against Women Act of 1993, which is modeled on the Civil Rights Act of 1964, states that domestic violence crimes violate a woman's civil rights and that she can sue the

offender for damages. The law prohibits a **batterer** from crossing state lines to commit domestic violence, and it orders that **restraining orders** be honored across state lines. A restraining order prohibits the abuser from contacting the victim (including making phone calls and sending letters) and requires the offender to stay away from the victim's home, school, or workplace. The federal act allocates money for programs to encourage arrest of batterers, train police, and educate law enforcement officials about domestic abuse. It also establishes and supports hotlines, shelters, and community programs that address violence against women. Some observers feel that the most important aspect of this law is that the federal government finally sent a statement that domestic violence should not be tolerated.

States also have laws against rape and other forms of sexual assault, and these laws apply to sexual abuse of spouses or partners. Until recently, however, men who raped their wives could not be prosecuted. Many people believed that a wife was required to submit to her husband in all matters, including sexual relations. In this view of marriage, a husband did not need his wife's consent to have sex with her. Today, men who rape their wives can be prosecuted, although it is still treated as a lesser crime than rape by a stranger. In some states, rape by a husband is a crime only if the couple is not living together.

Current laws dealing with divorce and child custody also address domestic violence. Most states now have laws that require the court to consider domestic violence in making custody decisions. Allowing a child to witness **battering** is considered child endangerment, which is a crime in some states. A person convicted of child endangerment may be considered an unfit guardian and lose custody of the child.

The perpetrator of domestic abuse may be charged with a **misdemeanor** or a **felony** offense. Both are crimes, but a felony is a more serious offense. The nature of the charge depends on the circumstances, whether a weapon was used, the age of the offender and the victim, and the extent of the injuries. For example, slapping or pushing one's spouse would likely be considered a misdemeanor if the victim was not seriously injured. By contrast, an assault with a deadly weapon such as a knife or gun would be considered a felony in most state. For many misdemeanors, the police must actually witness the crime. However, domestic violence laws allow the police to arrest a suspect if they have good reason to believe an assault occurred.

TEENS SPEAK

At First I Didn't Talk about the Violence Even to My Parents

I wasn't even sure it was abuse until I was listening to a call-in radio show for teens. A caller who is gay was talking about the way his boyfriend treated him. I thought, "I'm a girl, but that sounds just like the way my boyfriend treats me." He once pushed me out of the car because I wouldn't have sex with him. Another time, he shoved me against my locker. I was always lying to my friends and parents about my cuts and bruises.

After hearing that radio show, I told a school advisor about my boyfriend. She dismissed it until she saw my bruises. She said I should report what happened to the police. I didn't want to get my boyfriend into trouble, but then I got angry. He didn't seem to care that he was hurting me.

My parents and I went to the police. The police didn't want to pursue it because they said it was my word against his, but my parents insisted. We also talked to someone at the shelter for battered women. They told us that he needed help, and he needed to be stopped or he would continue to abuse other women. Luckily, he's still a minor so he went to juvenile court. I had to testify but the judge was nice. She believed me, and she told him he had to learn better ways to communicate. He looked at me with a lot of hate and I was scared. But she told him he had to stay away from me. She also sent him to a different school. I didn't follow all the legal talk but I think she said he would be on probation, and if he came anywhere near me she would send him to a juvenile facility.

LEGAL APPROACHES TO DOMESTIC ABUSE

Significant changes in the laws concerning domestic abuse have occurred since the 1970s when states began to recognize domestic violence as a crime. Before this time, law enforcement agencies looked upon domestic violence as a "family matter" that should be settled without legal intervention. However, according to law professor Edna

Erez, leaders of the feminist movement of the 1970s raised public awareness about the problem of domestic violence. Today domestic violence is an issue for the **criminal justice system** to prosecute and punish. The criminal justice system includes law enforcement officials such as local, state, and federal police; the court system including defense attorneys, prosecutors and judges; and the corrections system of jails, prisons, probation boards, and parole boards.

Arrest

Police are the first responders in the criminal justice system to incidents of domestic violence. Many states require that police make an arrest when they respond to a domestic violence call. However, as with many aspects of abuse legislation, the laws vary from one state to another. In some states, police officers who do not make arrests in response to domestic violence incidents must file a report explaining their decision. Nevertheless, some officers still view domestic abuse as a private matter between partners, particularly if the state does not have a mandatory (legally required) arrest policy. If police arrive and find both parties acting violently, they often arrest neither person, even though one partner may have been acting in self-defense.

If the **batterer** flees the scene when police are called, the police are supposed to search for the abuser immediately or write a report explaining why they did not try to do so. Police officers are also supposed to follow up the next day on efforts to locate the offender. In reality, they do not always do so, but some states hold the police responsible for the victim's safety if no arrest is made.

When the police make an arrest, they must read the alleged abuser his rights before taking him to jail. Unfortunately, the perpetrator may not remain in jail long following arrest, thus placing the victim in greater danger. Victims of domestic abuse should have an emergency plan in case an abusive partner continues the abuse upon being released from jail. The plan should include a safe place to stay if the victim feels unsafe at home.

Q & A

Question: How can I be sure my ex-boyfriend will be prosecuted for beating me up?

Answer: There are no guarantees. Most state domestic violence laws do not apply to dating violence. If he is a minor, the matter will probably be taken up in juvenile court. If you are a minor and he is not, he will be tried in criminal court if prosecuted. Juvenile court is usually less formal than criminal court. Responsible juvenile court judges will take the issue seriously and not simply see it as "teenage love" or simply suggest that the two of you stop seeing each other. The judge will probably send him to detention, release him to his parent's custody, sentence him to probation and/or order that he get treatment. Even if domestic violence laws do not cover dating violence, the state can charge him with other crimes, such as criminal harassment or assault.

Restraining orders

A victim who feels that an abuser presents a threat to his or her safety may ask the courts to issue a restraining order against the abuser. The order may require the offender to pay spousal support, child support, or payment for alternative housing for the victim. The protective order can also require counseling for the offender. If the treatment is completed, the charges against the offender may be dropped.

In some states the person seeking the restraining order must be married or related to the offender or have a child with him or her. In other states, the orders can be issued against an acquaintance. A small number of states issue restraining orders against someone with whom the person making the complaint has no relationship, such as when the person is stalking or constantly following him or her.

A court can issue a restraining order as a short-term emergency measure or as a long-term measure after a legal hearing. An emergency restraining order is issued if the person making the complaint is in danger of immediate harm. It is usually valid for only a few days until a hearing can be held with the alleged abuser present. After the hearing, a long-term restraining order may be issued. Long-term orders remain valid for as little as three months in some states and up to three years in others. However, batterers do not necessarily honor restraining orders. Angered by the arrest and restraint order, they may become even more of a danger to the victim. An offender who violates a restraining order can be arrested on a misdemeanor or felony charge.

Prosecution

Prosecution is the decision by the state to bring legal charges against an alleged criminal. Prosecution can result in a court trial or an out of-court settlement. A case that goes to trial can result in dismissal of the case, a guilty or not guilty verdict, or mandatory treatment for the abuser. In an out-of-court settlement, the defendant typically agrees to admit responsibility in return for receiving a lighter punishment.

Prosecutors are the lawyers for the government. They are called district attorneys; state, county or city attorneys; or prosecutors. They are responsible for presenting court cases against batterers and obtaining convictions. Prosecutors have some leeway concerning the charges and punishments they seek for batterers. Some states have the option of sending abusers arrested for the first time to treatment programs instead of (or in addition to) jail.

Unfortunately, many victims are unwilling to prosecute their abusers. In some cases they fear the abuser will not be punished or will serve only a short sentence, then return home to continue the abuse. In other cases, the victim may be reluctant to send a spouse or loved one to jail for emotional or financial reasons. Despite these reservations, however, offenders must be prosecuted for the system to effectively protect victims of abuse.

Because so many victims withdraw their charges after an arrest, many jurisdictions have adopted laws that allow the state to prosecute a batterer even if the victim does not press charges. The victim's cooperation is still important in obtaining a conviction, though. In some places, **victim advocates** help victims negotiate the criminal justice system and understand the importance of obtaining a conviction. Some police departments are also training officers how to investigate cases of abuse so they can be proven without the victim's testimony.

Fact Or Fiction?

Arresting batterers or issuing civil protection orders are useless in preventing abuse.

Fact: Most experts agree that actions by one part of the criminal justice system are only effective when the rest of the system works. That is, police must make arrests, prosecutors must bring charges against the accused, and judges must sentence convicted batterers to prison, treatment programs, and/or probation with monitoring. It is important for batterers to receive the message from the community that domestic violence will not be tolerated and that the criminal justice and law enforcement systems will intercede until the violence ends.

Incarceration

One form of punishment for a convicted abuser is incarceration, or time in prison. Judges have the discretion to sentence first offenders to **probation** if they feel the defendant is unlikely to repeat the abusive behavior. They may also sentence repeat offenders to longer prison sentences. In some states, jail time is mandatory for felony battering. Some battered women's advocates, however, believe that laws requiring jail time cause as many problems as they solve. They argue that batterers are less likely to plead guilty if they face the prospect of prison time. In addition, victims who do not want their spouses or partners serving time in jail may be less likely to participate in the prosecution. In these cases, the batterer is more likely to go free—and continue the abuse.

Many of the people who batter have no criminal record and hold a job. The judicial system often considers such individuals less likely to repeat their offenses and therefore sentences them to probation. However, offenders who serve no jail time may still need special monitoring to protect their victims. For this reason, courts in some states require batterers to wear electronic monitoring devices when they are released on bail or following a release from jail after conviction.

CHILD ABUSE LAWS

Child abuse is the use of physical, emotional, or verbal violence to control the behavior of a child. To meet the legal definition of child abuse, the violence must be committed by **caregivers** such as parents, guardians, other adults in the home, baby-sitters, chaperones, or other adults permanently or temporarily responsible for a child's care. An adult can also be found guilty of child abuse if he or she was legally responsible for the child and failed to protect the child from abuse by another person. Violence toward a child perpetrated by other adults is also a criminal act, but it is considered assault, not child abuse.

Child abuse laws deal not only with physical abuse but also with emotional abuse, such as subjecting a child to extreme public humiliation. Failure to provide for the child's basic needs, known as **neglect**, is against the law in every state. Parents or legal guardians who fail to meet a child's basic needs for food, clothing, medical care, and supervision are guilty of neglect.

In every state, people in certain professions are required by law to report suspected child abuse. These individuals, known as **mandated adults**, include doctors, nurses, dentists, mental health professionals, social workers, teachers, day care workers, and law enforcement personnel. In some states, clergy, foster parents, attorneys, and camp counselors also are required to report abuse. Some states require anyone who suspects child abuse to report it to law enforcement authorities. People can report suspected child abuse through special hotlines. Most states protect people from being sued if it turns out the suspicions were wrong and no abuse occurred.

Each state has a system of family courts that deal with cases of child abuse and determine whether the victim may safely remain with his or her parents. The court can take a child away from a parent

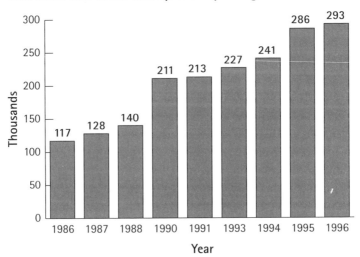

DID YOU KNOW?

Increased Reporting of Elder Abuse

According to the National Center on Elder Abuse (NCEA), the number of cases of elder abuse reported in the United States increased by more than 250 percent between 1986 and 1996. The NCEA says that much of the increase is due to greater awareness and more widespread reporting of elder abuse.

Source: National Center on Elder Abuse, 1997.

because of abuse or neglect but usually seeks to reunite the family after problems have been addressed. A family court judge may recommend parenting classes, substance abuse treatment, or other efforts he or she feels are needed to reduce the chances of future abuse. The child typically remains in foster care or with other relatives during this time. If the parent makes little effort to improve or does not complete the recommended programs, the state may end his or her parental rights—not a step the state takes lightly or quickly. However, if an individual loses parental rights to a child, another family may then adopt the child.

ELDER ABUSE LAWS

Elder abuse is the use of physical, emotional, or verbal violence to control a dependent elderly person. The federal Older Americans Act (OAA) defines elder abuse and provides federal funds for elder abuse awareness, training, and coordination activities in states and local communities. The 1992 Title VII Vulnerable Elder Rights Protection Act updated the OAA and included funding for states to investigate and prosecute elder abuse.

Every state has laws that create a system for reporting and investigating elder abuse, and for providing social services to help victims and prevent further abuse. In most states these laws are not limited to older persons but apply to any abused adult who is considered disabled, impaired, or vulnerable by state law. State laws vary widely in many areas including:

- The definition of abuse
- The types of abuse, neglect, and exploitation covered by law
- Whether the abuse is considered a criminal or civil offense
- Who, if anyone, is required to report abuse
- Who is responsible for investigating abuse
- The age at which a victim is eligible to receive protection or social services
- The circumstances under which a victim is eligible to receive protection or social services
- Remedies for abuse and strategies to prevent future abuse

Some state laws apply only to individuals who reside in the community, while others include individuals who reside in long-term care facilities, such as nursing homes. Each state defines a long-term care facility differently. Some also include other types of institutions, such as mental health facilities, in their statutes. In states where the law only covers those who reside in the community, a separate law addresses institutional abuse. These laws create a system for reporting, investigating, and dealing with elder abuse in long-term care facilities or other facilities specified by the law.

In some states, the laws defining and punishing elder abuse are becoming more like those that deal with criminal acts committed against strangers. Some states now allow elder abuse to be prosecuted as a criminal act. A growing number of states are also passing laws that call for specific criminal penalties for various forms of elder abuse. Others have begun to define certain types of elder abuse, such as sexual abuse, in the same words used in state criminal laws. Even without laws targeted specifically at elder abuse, abusers can be prosecuted under basic criminal laws including those dealing with battery, assault, theft, fraud, rape, manslaughter, or murder.

Other legal tools are also in place to help senior citizens suffering from abuse. For example, domestic violence or family violence laws may provide for restraining orders in cases of physical abuse against elders. The 1992 Title VII Vulnerable Elder Rights Protection Act also requires every state to establish a Long-Term Care Ombudsman Program (LTCOP). The ombudsman is responsible for acting on behalf of residents in long-term care facilities who experience abuse, violation of their rights, or other problems. States that do not establish LTCOPs are ineligible to receive federal funds under the Older Americans Act.

The LTCOPs are a key part of state efforts to end elder abuse in institutions. The ombudsman responds to complaints of abuse in long-term care facilities. If evidence of abuse is found, the LTCOP notifies law enforcement agencies, the state agency responsible for licensing and certifying long-term care facilities, or an adult protective services program that will act to protect the victim from further abuse. In some states the LTCOP itself has the authority to investigate and respond to abuse in long-term care facilities.

State and federal laws against domestic abuse, child abuse, and elder abuse send the message that these activities are crimes that need to be addressed and prosecuted. Issues that were once considered private matters that should be left to the family are now recognized as problems that concern the larger society. By taking legal steps to prevent and punish abuse, states have embraced their obligation to protect the most vulnerable members of the community.

See also: Abuse in Society; Child Abuse; Child Sexual Abuse; Domestic Partner Abuse; Elder Abuse

FURTHER READING

American Prosecutors Research Institute. *Investigation and Prosecution of Child Abuse.* Thousand Oaks, CA: Sage Publications, 2003.

Brownell, Patricia J. *Family Crimes against the Elderly: Elder Abuse and the Criminal Justice System.* Hamden, CT: Garland Publishing, 1998.

Sagatun, Inger, and Leonard Edwards. *Child Abuse and the Legal System.* Belmont, CA: Wadsworth Publishing Company, 1995.

Schlesinger Buzawa, Eva, and Carl G. Buzawa. *Domestic Violence: The Criminal Justice Response, Third Edition.* Thousand Oaks, CA: Sage Publications, 2002.

■ MEDIA AND ABUSE

Forms of mass communication such as newspapers, magazines, radio, or television. The media have played an important role in raising awareness of and shaping public perceptions about abuse. Many observers credit the media for publicizing the problem of abuse, thus removing the veil of shame and secrecy that prevented an honest discussion of it. The media's approach to the subject of abuse, however, is not entirely positive. Critics point out that media coverage often presents a distorted, sensationalized view of abuse.

PUBLICIZING ABUSE

Champions of the media suggest that news reporting has been an important factor in focusing public attention on the issue of abuse. For example, the 1996 article "Defining the Problem" in the journal *Child Abuse & Neglect* argued that the media have been essential to societal awareness of child abuse and neglect. The article stated that news reporting on specific cases of abuse as well as on research and intervention was more important than community education campaigns in publicizing the issue of child abuse.

While breakthrough studies about abuse appear first in professional journals, they often come to public attention through news reports in the popular media. In the 1984 book *Making an Issue of Child Abuse: Political Agenda-Setting for Social Problems,* Barbara Nelson, dean of the School of Public Policy and Social Research at the University of California–Los Angeles, points out that media reaction to the first major study of child abuse was key in "transforming the once minor charity concern called 'cruelty to children' into an important social welfare issue." She notes that the 1962 article "The Battered Child Syndrome" in the *Journal of the American Medical Association* generated a flood of stories in popular magazines such as *Time.* Nelson argues that these stories were as important as the study itself "in creating the sense of an urgent national problem."

A 2002 report "Coverage in Context: How Thoroughly the News Media Report Five Key Children's Issues" suggests that the media still devote considerable coverage to issues of child abuse. The report studied three months of news reporting on issues including youth crime/violence, child abuse/neglect, teen childbearing, child care, and child health insurance coverage. Two of the five—youth crime/violence and child abuse/neglect—received "extensive" news coverage, accounting for nine out of every 10 news stories about children presented during the three-month period.

According to some critics, other forms of abuse have not been covered as thoroughly as child abuse. A 2000 study by the Berkeley Media Studies Group titled "Distracted by Drama: How California Newspapers Portray Intimate Partner Violence" found that the media consistently underreport domestic violence. According to the study, other forms of violence received between six and 10 times more coverage in California newspapers than did domestic partner violence. The 2002 survey "Coverage of Domestic Violence Fatalities by Newspapers in Washington State" found that stories about such fatalities typically fail to mention the fact that the death was due to domestic violence. Fewer than 10 percent of the 230 newspaper articles included in the survey reported the incident as domestic violence.

MEDIA PRESENTATION OF ABUSE

While the media receives mixed reviews on the amount of coverage it gives to issues of abuse, it is widely criticized for the way it presents those issues. Even many who credit the media with spotlighting abuse feel that news coverage often conveys an inaccurate and incomplete picture of the dynamics of abuse. Critics of the media claim that such portrayals hinder community efforts to prevent abuse.

Perhaps the most frequent criticism of media presentations of abuse is the charge of sensationalism. Critics claim that news reports about abuse tend to focus on the most shocking or sensational aspects of a case. For example, the study "Distracted by Drama" found that newspaper coverage of domestic violence was much more "murder-oriented" than coverage of other types of violence. Stories about domestic violence were five to 10 times more likely to feature a homicide than stories about other forms of violence. The study also showed that the media portrayed domestic violence–related murders as being much more common than is actually the case. In the newspapers surveyed by the study, more than 60 percent of the domestic violence stories were about homicides, even though only a small fraction of local arrests for domestic violence involved murder charges.

Such concerns about media sensationalism are not new. The conclusions of a 1980 study titled "Magazine Coverage" showed that news stories about child sexual abuse and pornography have long been covered in a very sensationalistic manner. The article, which appeared in the book *Child Abuse: An Agenda for Action*, reported that magazine coverage of incest was particularly marked by sensationalism. The study argued that reporters and editors were torn between desires to "cover serious social issues" and "continuing to turn a profit."

Fact Or Fiction?

Newspaper reports of domestic violence typically blame the victim for the abuse or make excuses for the perpetrator.

Fact: The 2000 study "Distracted by Drama: How California Newspapers Portray Intimate Partner Violence" found that reports of domestic violence rarely blamed the victims or excused the perpetrators of domestic violence. Fewer than 4 percent of the articles surveyed in the study blamed the victims for their abuse. However, the study also discovered that news stories blamed domestic violence victims for their abuse more often than victims of other types of violent crime.

LACK OF CONTEXT

The media are also frequently criticized for failing to place stories of abuse in a context that makes the information relevant for the public at large. "Distracted by Drama" faults the media for portraying abuse as a personal or family problem instead of a widespread social problem. Focusing on the most bizarre or shocking aspects of a story makes abuse seem like something that could not possibly happen in a "normal" family or relationship. This approach makes it much more difficult for the public at large to identify with and acknowledge the seriousness of the problem. A lack of public awareness or concern undermines efforts to deal with and prevent the spread of abuse.

The 2002 report "Coverage in Context" also faults the media for omitting important information in the coverage of abuse. The study reported that fewer than 5 percent of all stories about child abuse and neglect helped readers understand how this related to wider trends in

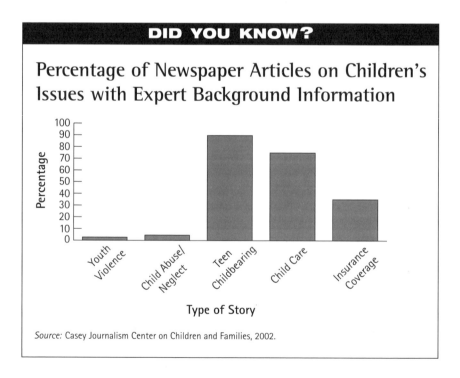

DID YOU KNOW?

Percentage of Newspaper Articles on Children's Issues with Expert Background Information

Type of Story

Source: Casey Journalism Center on Children and Families, 2002.

society. Only about 34 percent of the stories provided any general background information on the issues of child abuse or neglect.

The 2000 Boston College Media Research Action Project found that media reports of abuse suffered from both lack of context and inaccurate information about the nature of domestic violence. According the study, which surveyed 88 newspaper articles about domestic violence fatalities, fewer than 20 percent of the articles linked the murders to domestic violence. Fewer than half of the stories presented information about domestic violence statistics, the dynamics of abuse, or community resources for victims of abuse.

INACCURACY AND STEREOTYPES

Several studies have also charged that media coverage of abuse perpetuates inaccurate stereotypes about the abuser, the victim, and the dynamics of abusive relationships. Almost half (48 percent) of the articles surveyed in the 2002 study "Coverage of Domestic Violence Fatalities by Newspapers in Washington State" suggested an excuse for the abuser's behavior. Some 17 percent of the stories contained language that seemed to blame the victim for the violence. For example, one article quoted a relative as saying the victim "had a habit of getting involved with men who abused her."

Another myth about domestic violence frequently repeated in the stories surveyed by the Washington study was that abusers are easy to identify. Interviews with shocked neighbors who described perpetrators as "clean-cut" or "well-rounded," suggest that domestic abuse is committed only by seedy looking, disreputable characters. In reality, abusers come from all social classes or walks of life. The Boston College Media Research Action Project cited other myths about abuse that were reinforced by media coverage, including:

- Domestic violence is something that happens to somebody else.
- Substance abuse is responsible for domestic violence.
- Domestic violence homicides are unpredictable tragedies rather then the inevitable outcome of a long-term pattern of abuse.
- Domestic violence is a tragic expression of love, rather than an act of control.

According to some studies, part of the reason for the media's distorted coverage of abuse can be traced to the sources used by reporters. The Washington newspaper study found that in 40 of the 44 cases of domestic homicides covered by the papers, reporters did not consult a single expert on domestic violence before writing their stories. Police reports and comments were the most frequently consulted sources. The study by Stanford University's Dart Center reached similar conclusions. Researchers found that other victims of abuse and therapists who counsel abuse victims were rarely quoted in news reports about domestic violence.

IMPACT OF MEDIA COVERAGE

Media coverage of abuse has had practical effects beyond simply raising awareness about the subject of abuse. A 2001 report in the journal *Child Abuse Prevention Issues* titled "Child Abuse and the Media" suggests that media coverage has been critical to the passage of anti-abuse legislation in several nations. The article cites the extensive media attention given to a 1993 case of child abuse in Australia. Several Australian newspapers not only gave prominent daily coverage to the case but also began a public campaign to promote new laws about reporting child abuse. The laws, which received little public attention or support before the media focus on the case, passed soon afterward. One comment described the phenomenon as "legislation by tabloid."

Media coverage of abuse has also led to increasing public criticism of child welfare systems in the United States and elsewhere. "Child abuse and the media" cited a number of studies showing that increased media attention on child abuse has resulted in a backlash against perceived inefficiency and incompetence in the agencies responsible for protecting children. One of those studies, a 1994 report titled "The Literature of the Backlash" found that reporting was increasingly critical of the child protection system. According to the study, the media frequently alleges that the child protection system is "out of control" and has major problems. It often portrays child protection as a "witch hunt" and blames child protection professionals for contributing to hysteria about child abuse. Professionals are often portrayed as the problem rather than contributing to the solution.

IMPROVING MEDIA COVERAGE

To assist reporters in providing readers with accurate, balanced, and, meaningful information about abuse, the Washington State Coalition

Against Domestic Violence published a guide titled "Covering Domestic Violence." The guide includes the following tips for accurately covering domestic violence.

- Acknowledge that domestic violence is a widespread community problem, not a private matter.
- Research the perpetrator's prior history of violent behavior and cover the crime in the context of domestic violence rather than as an unexplained tragedy.
- Explain that violence often occurs when a victim tries to leave an abusive relationship.
- Explain to readers the warning signs of an abusive relationship such as excessive jealousy or unexplained injuries on the victim.

The guide also offers tips on what to avoid when covering domestic violence stories.

- Do not call domestic abuse a "relationship problem"; it is a violent crime and should be described as such.
- Do not focus on the victim's behavior, as this tends to place blame on the victim; also avoid language that tends to blame the victim.
- Do not assume that members of some ethnic groups or social classes are violent and others are not; point out that anyone can be an abuser.
- Avoid using as sources people who are emotionally connected to the perpetrator or people who do not have significant information about the crime or those involved.
- Do not treat domestic violence as something that cannot be solved by community action.

The media has been indispensable to raising awareness of abuse, but it clearly has much to do to improve the way it covers issues of abuse. Fortunately, media observers have not only identified the major errors made by the media but also offered solutions to some of these problems in coverage. However, the media still must act on those suggestions while at the same time balancing their concerns for accurate reporting with the need to sell their product to the public.

See also: Abusers, Common Traits of; Child Abuse; Domestic Partner Abuse; Homicide; Legal Intervention

FURTHER READING
Cote, William E., and Roger Simpson. *Covering Violence.* New York: Columbia University Press, 2000.
Franklin, Bob. *Social Policy, the Media and Misrepresentation.* London: Routledge, 1999.
Meyers, Marian. *News Coverage of Violence against Women.* Thousand Oaks, CA: Sage Publications, 1996.

■ MEN AND ABUSE

Many people believe that the vast majority of those who commit abuse are males. After all, men are generally larger and stronger than women and, according to the Department of Justice, in 2001 men committed about 88 percent of all violent crime in the United States. However, men are frequently the victims of domestic partner abuse, and they seem to be less likely than women to commit some other forms of abuse. Clearly, men are not always the perpetrators or aggressors when it comes to abuse.

MEN AS PERPETRATORS

The answer to the question of which sex commits abuse more often depends upon the type of abuse one considers. For example, men are much more likely to be perpetrators of domestic violence than are women. However, they are less likely to abuse children and no more likely than women to abuse the elderly.

Domestic partner abuse

Intimate Partner Violence, a 2000 publication by the Department of Justice, reported that women were five times more likely than men to be victims of domestic violence. The study revealed that spouses or partners killed 33 percent of all female murder victims in the United States in 1998. According to the National Institute of Justice and the Centers for Disease Control and Prevention, a current or former domestic partner victimized 75 percent of the women age 18 and over who were raped or physically assaulted.

Some people argue that these statistics overstate the differences between males and females when it comes to committing domestic abuse. Indeed, other surveys suggest that men commit a smaller percentage of domestic abuse than reported by the Department of Justice. According to the 2001 National Violence Against Women Survey (NVAWS), women were victims of 64.4 percent of all incidents of domestic abuse in the United States, while men were victims in 35.6 percent of all incidents. Of the women surveyed by the NVAWS, 24.8 percent had been raped or physically assaulted by a spouse or partner. Although that is more than three times the rate for men (7.6 percent), it is still considerably smaller than the difference reported by the Department of Justice.

Several studies from the 1970s and 1980s showed even smaller differences between rates of male and female domestic abuse. "Fatal Violence among Spouses in the United States," a 1989 article in the *Journal of Public Health*, reported that from 1976 to 1985 husbands murdered their wives about 30 percent more often than wives murdered their husbands. In the 1986 article "Societal Change and Change in Family Violence from 1976 to 1985 as Revealed by Two National Surveys," the *Journal of Marriage and the Family* reported that the number of female victims of domestic violence in the United States declined from 12.1 percent to 11.3 percent. During the same time period, the number of male victims increased from 11.6 percent to 12.1 percent. In a report on teen dating, the November 1986 issue of the journal *Social Work* found that girls were more frequently violent than boys.

More recent research in this area has shown mixed results. For example, a 2000 review of studies published in *Psychological Bulletin* titled "Sex Differences in Aggression between Heterosexual Partners: A Meta-analytic Review" found that women were more likely than men to use acts of physical aggression. "Adolescent Dating Violence. Do Adolescents Follow in their Friends' or Their Parents' Footsteps?" a 2004 study in the *Journal of Interpersonal Violence*, reported very small sex differences in dating abuse, with females engaging in violence slightly more often than males. However, a 2002 article in the *Journal of Interpersonal Violence* titled "A Multivariate Analysis of Risk Markers for Dating Violence Victimization" found no difference in physical violence between men and women in dating relationships.

These and other studies indicate that women are as likely as men to use physical violence in intimate relationships. So why are men seen as more violent? One reason is that men tend to inflict more—and more serious—injuries than do females. Although the article "Sex Differences in Aggression between Heterosexual Partners" reported that women engage in intimate violence slightly more often than men, it also found that women were more likely to be injured by domestic partner violence. "Marital Aggression: Impact, Injury, and Health Correlates for Husbands and Wives," a 1992 article published in the *Archives of Internal Medicine* found that half of women but only about one-third of men suffered injuries as a result of domestic violence, even though the rate of violence was roughly the same for both sexes.

Fact Or Fiction?

Men who are happy in their relationships do not hit their partners.

Fact: Battering is rarely caused by dissatisfaction in the relationship. Many batterers value their relationship and are driven by fear of losing it. They are insecure, dependent, and jealous to the point of suspecting every move their partners make. Their use of violence is not about helping the relationship; it is about controlling their partners. Abusers typically do not know how to communicate or handle their feelings. They try to exert power and control in the relationship in order to maintain it.

Child and elder abuse

Unlike domestic abuse, men commit **child abuse** much less frequently than women. The Department of Health and Human Services' Administration for Children, Youth, and Families (ACF) reported in 2002 that 40.3 percent of all child abuse was perpetrated by the mother alone, and that women were responsible for 62.3 of all cases of child abuse. Males, by comparison, were involved in 37.7 percent of child abuse violations.

Men and women also engage in different forms of child abuse. The ACF reports that males are much more likely to sexually abuse children than are women. Almost three-quarters (74.1 percent) of cases of child sexual abuse were committed by men. By contrast, men were much less likely to **neglect** children in their care. Just 26.1 percent of child neglect cases involved male perpetrators. Men and women were about equally likely to engage in **physical abuse** and **psychological abuse** of children.

Government statistics show that men are slightly less likely than women to commit **elder abuse**. The National Center on Elder Abuse found that, in 1996, men committed 47.4 percent of all cases of elder abuse in the United States. However, as with child abuse, men are responsible for the overwhelming majority of cases of **sexual abuse** of elders. Experts suggest that sex differences in child abuse and elder abuse relate to opportunity rather than a natural tendency toward violence. Because women are more often caretakers for children and the elderly, they have many more opportunities to commit abuse against these populations.

MEN AS VICTIMS

A good deal of controversy surrounds the issue of men as victims of abuse. Society typically portrays men as perpetrators of physical abuse, not as victims. However, the studies cited earlier indicate that men are victims, while also raising questions about just how often it happens and how serious it is compared to abuse of women. Some studies suggest that women commit violence against their partners as often as men do. However, the injuries to men are not usually as severe and are not reported as often to law enforcement authorities.

Official government statistics reflect the view of men as perpetrators rather than victims. According to the Bureau of Justice Statistics (BJS), in 1998 women reported 876,340 cases of abuse in the United States, while men were victims in 157,330 reports. The BJS also found that domestic abuse accounted for 22 percent of all violent crime against women, but only 3 percent of violent crime against men. As noted earlier, some researchers have challenged whether these statistics reflect the true extent of female-on-male domestic violence.

Although males were injured less often than females during domestic violence incidents, they were more often assaulted with weapons or other objects. The 2002 National Violence Against Women Survey reported that 59.5 percent of women who engaged in domestic violence threw something at their intended victim, compared to 36.7 percent of males. Men were almost twice as likely to be hit with an object (43.2 percent to 22.6 percent for women) or threatened with a knife (21.6 percent to 12.7 percent), and more than twice as likely to be assaulted with a knife (10.8 percent to 4.1 percent).

Q & A

Question: I think my best friend's girlfriend is abusing him. What can I do?

Answer: Remember that abuse is about power and control. Is she using put-downs, mind games, and other verbal or emotional methods to control him? Does she try to keep him from spending time with you and other friends and family? Does she threaten or intimidate him? Talk to him about your concerns. Be respectful, and don't tease him. It is difficult for males to admit to being either physically or emotionally abused by a female. If he does recognize her behavior as abusive, encourage him to talk to an adult who might be familiar with the problem of battered males.

According to a 1997 study by the Department of Health and Human Services, 48 percent of child abuse victims were male. The study found that boys were more likely than girls to suffer from neglect, physical abuse, or failure to receive medical attention. The study also reported that three times as many girls as boys were victims of child sexual abuse. Even so, a 1996 review of studies of child abuse titled "Sexual Abuse of Males: Prevalence, Possible Lasting Effects, and Resources" found that approximately one in every six boys is sexually abused before the age of 16.

A 1994 article in the *Journal of Traumatic Stress* titled "The Psychological Impact of Sexual Abuse: Content Analysis of Interviews with Male Survivors" outlined some of the lasting effects of childhood sexual abuse on adult males. These include:

- Anxiety
- Depression
- Hostility and anger
- Low self-esteem
- Relationship problems
- Sexual problems
- Sleep disturbances
- Thoughts of suicide

The article also linked childhood sexual abuse to confusion about sexual orientation in adulthood, fear and hatred of homosexuals, having multiple sexual partners, and violent behavior.

Despite evidence that men are frequently the victims of domestic and dating violence, few services exist for **battered** men. While communities with large gay populations are beginning to offer services for battered gay men, straight men battered by women find little help. In addition, men are reluctant to seek help from police, the courts, or social services because of the stigma of being abused by a woman. The best chance for most male victims of abuse to receive help is by contacting a private therapist. However, therapy is expensive and does not offer the immediate help that a shelter or other community-based resources can provide.

See also: Abuse in Society; Child Abuse; Child Sexual Abuse; Dating Abuse; Domestic Partner Abuse; Elder Abuse; Women and Abuse

FURTHER READING
Bancroft, Lundy. *Why Does He Do That? Inside the Minds of Angry and Controlling Men.* New York: G. P. Putnam's Sons, 2002.
Cook, Philip W. *Abused Men.* New York: Praeger Publishers, 1997.
Harway, Michele. What Causes Men's Violence against Women? Thousand Oaks, CA: Sage Publications, 1999.
Tobin, Rod. Alone and Forgotten: The Sexually Abused Man. Ottawa, ON: Creative Bound Press, 1999.

■ MENTAL HEALTH AND ABUSE
See: Abuse in Society; Child Abuse; Child Sexual Abuse; Elder Abuse; Post-traumatic Stress Disorder and Abuse; Psychological Abuse

■ NEGLECT AS ABUSE
See: Child Abuse; Women and Abuse

■ POVERTY AND ABUSE
See: Abuse, Theories of; Domestic Partner Abuse

■ POST-TRAUMATIC STRESS DISORDER AND ABUSE
A psychological disorder that can occur as a result of experiencing or witnessing an extremely stressful event. A variety of situations can

trigger post-traumatic stress disorder (PTSD), such as military combat, natural disasters, serious accidents, and violent personal assaults—including incidents of domestic violence. According to the National Center for Post-Traumatic Stress Disorder (NCPTSD), a victim may develop PTSD in response to any event perceived as potentially life-threatening. Persons suffering from PTSD may suffer severe psychological and emotional problems that can impair their ability to lead a normal life.

SYMPTOMS AND INCIDENCE OF PTSD

PTSD can trigger a host of harmful symptoms including:

- Reliving the event through flashbacks and nightmares
- Difficulty sleeping
- Feelings of detachment from the outside world
- Aggressive behavior
- High levels of daily stress
- Intense emotional reactions to anything seen as a threat

The NCPTSD reports that PTSD frequently occurs along with disorders such as substance abuse, **depression**, memory problems, and impairment of thinking and problem-solving skills. These additional disorders can complicate the problems suffered by victims of PTSD. Together, PTSD and related disorders can cause difficulty in family and social life, job instability, and problems dealing with responsibilities such as parenting.

According to the NCPTSD, 60.7 percent of men and 51.2 percent of women in the United States report that they have experienced at least one traumatic event, and most develop some of the symptoms of PTSD in the days immediately following the experience. However, only a small fraction develops PTSD. About 8 percent of men and about 20 percent of women show longer-term symptoms of PTSD. Some 30 percent of the people whose symptoms last more than a few days will suffer from PTSD for the rest of their lives. The NCPTSD estimates that about 7.8 percent of Americans suffer from PTSD at some time in their lives, and some 3.6 percent suffer from it in any given year. Women are twice as likely as men to develop PTSD. For most victims, PTSD is marked by periods in which the individual suffers from symptoms followed by periods in which he or she is relatively symptom-free. A minority of PTSD victims, however, suffer continuously from severe symptoms.

Q & A

Question: I've heard about Vietnam veterans suffering from PTSD, but never about its effects on veterans of other wars. Is PTSD something that has only recently been diagnosed by doctors?

Answer: PTSD is far from a new disorder. Ancient writers mentioned PTSD symptoms in men returning from battle. The first medical record of PTSD occurred in the Civil War, where the condition was called DaCosta's Syndrome. Doctors from World War II recorded descriptions of combat veterans and Holocaust survivors treated immediately after the war who showed signs of PTSD. However, in-depth research into PTSD did not start until after the Vietnam War. This is why so many Vietnam veterans have been identified as suffering from PTSD compared to the surviving veterans of other wars.

PTSD AND DOMESTIC VIOLENCE

A number of research studies have demonstrated that witnesses and victims of domestic partner abuse and child abuse often develop symptoms of PTSD. According to a 1996 report by the American Academy of Experts in Traumatic Stress titled "Effects of Domestic Violence on Children and Adolescents: An Overview," a person repeatedly exposed to domestic violence may develop PTSD. The article reports that more than half of the school-age children in domestic violence shelters show evidence of PTSD. The report's conclusions are supported by the results of other research examining the link between domestic violence and PTSD. A 2004 article in the journal *Psychiatric News*, titled "PTSD, Other Disorders Evident in Kids Who Witness Domestic Violence" found that children exposed to domestic violence are twice as likely to develop PTSD and related disorders as children who are not exposed to violence.

However, it is not only the victims or witnesses of domestic abuse and child abuse who may suffer from PTSD. Some studies have found that persons who suffer from PTSD may be particularly likely to abuse their partners or children. A 1997 article in the journal *NCP Clinical Quarterly* titled "Post-traumatic Stress Disorder and the Perpetration of Domestic Violence" outlined a number of striking similarities in behavior between combat veterans who suffer from PTSD and men who commit domestic violence. Both groups showed greater than average rates of substance abuse and depression, a general tendency toward aggressive behavior, higher general levels of stress than others in the population, and intense emotional reactions such as fear, anger, or guilt in response to threats. The article also reported that severe symptoms of PTSD are related to increased incidences of domestic violence by combat veterans.

A 1985 study in the *Journal of Consulting and Clinical Psychology* titled "Problems in Families of Male Vietnam Veterans with Post-traumatic Stress Disorders: Studies of Combat Veterans" found that 33 percent of Vietnam veterans with PTSD assaulted their partners in the previous year. By contrast, 15 percent of veterans without PTSD assaulted their partners during the same period. According to paper presented at the Fourth International Family Violence Research Conference in 1995 titled "The Cycle of Trauma: Marital Violence in Vietnam Veterans with PTSD," 63 percent of veterans with PTSD had assaulted their partners in the previous year, compared to 23 percent of veterans without PTSD. While none of these studies suggests that PTSD causes domestic violence, researchers do point out that PTSD can increase the likelihood of violence, especially if it is accompanied by other disorders such as substance abuse or depression.

Fact Or Fiction?

Childhood abuse can cause changes in the brain that affect one's thinking and behavior patterns.

Fact: According to the NCPTSD, prolonged exposure to abuse as a child can result in significant brain and hormonal changes. In this condition, called Complex PTSD, a child may experience difficulty with memory, learning, and controlling impulses and emotions. Brain changes may also lead to behavior problems, including aggressiveness, acting out sexually, alcohol or drug abuse, eating disorders, and self-destructive behaviors.

People suffering from Complex PTSD have difficulty controlling intense emotions such as anger, panic, or depression and may also experience mental disorders such as disorganized thought patterns, amnesia, or dissociation, a condition in which one feels detached from the outside world. Those who suffer from Complex PTSD as children are often diagnosed with mood or personality disorders as adults. Treatment of Complex PTSD typically takes much longer, progresses at a slower pace, and requires a much more sensitive and structured treatment environment than normal PTSD.

TREATING PTSD

Psychologists have developed a variety of approaches to treating victims of PTSD. These include various forms of **psychotherapy** as well as medication-based treatments. Some of the most commonly used approaches include cognitive-behavioral therapy (CBT), group therapy, brief psychodynamic therapy, eye movement desensitization and reprocessing (EMDR), and pharmacotherapy.

The goal of CBT is to change undesirable behaviors or emotions by changing the ways a person thinks and feels in situations that cause those behaviors. This approach involves several techniques including exposure therapy, in which the patient is encouraged to imagine the traumatic event that triggered the PTSD. By reliving the episode with the client, the therapist can help the patient gain control of the overwhelming fear and distress he or she experienced during the event. Some victims are not able to confront the trauma immediately, so the therapist may start with relaxation techniques to reduce the level of stress or addressing a small part of the overall event. CBT also helps the patient learn how to cope with anxiety and negative thoughts, manage his or her anger, and deal more constructively with stressful situations.

In group therapy, patients with PTSD meet to discuss their problems with other sufferers. Group members share stories of their experiences and the feelings of shame, anger, guilt, and fear they face as a result. Group therapy is based on the idea that individuals are more likely to open up and share their experiences and feelings in the presence of a supportive group of **peers**.

Brief psychodynamic therapy focuses less on the traumatic event itself than on the emotional problems caused by the experience. The patient is encouraged to recall the traumatic event and identify current situations in his or her life that set off painful memories and increase the severity of PTSD symptoms. The goal of brief psychodynamic therapy is to help the patient develop a greater sense of self-esteem and find more effective ways of thinking about and coping with stress and intense emotions.

EMDR combines elements of CBT and exposure therapy with techniques (such as hand claps or other sounds) used to draw the patient's attention back and forth from one side to the other. The therapy is based on research suggesting that alternating one's attention back and forth may make it easier for a patient to recover and process traumatic memories.

Pharmacotherapy, also known as drug therapy, is used to treat some cases of PTSD. Several types of **antidepressant drugs** are used in pharmacotherapy, but none by itself has proven effective in treating PTSD. Rather, the aim of most pharmacotherapy is to relieve the most severe symptoms of PTSD, particularly those that may interfere with the patient's ability to benefit from other forms of therapy. Once medications have controlled the worst symptoms of PTSD, the patient can begin psychotherapy to deal with issues of long-term recovery.

Despite these different approaches to treating PTSD, all of these therapies have much in common. For example, treatment only begins after the patient has been safely removed from the stressful situation. Therapy typically begins by educating survivors and their families about PTSD: what it is, what causes it, how it effects the victim and his or her loved ones, and the problems commonly associated with PTSD. All of these techniques also require that the patient relive the event in a safe environment while carefully examining his or her reactions to the event. Each approach also focuses on dealing with the strong emotions related to the event. Finally, the various methods teach the patient to cope with the memories, which usually do completely go away. The idea is to learn how to manage one's reactions to the memories when they do occur.

The studies that demonstrate links between post-traumatic stress disorder and abuse emphasize just how serious and long-lasting the damage from domestic violence or child abuse can be. PTSD is a disorder commonly caused by the shock of combat or the devastation of natural disasters, yet family violence and abuse can produce the same intense fear and adverse psychological reactions among its victims. This painful reality is part of the tragic legacy of abuse.

See also: Child Abuse; Domestic Partner Abuse; Psychological Abuse

FURTHER READING
Eth, Spencer, and Gerald Kay, eds. *PTSD in Children and Adolescents.* Washington, DC: American Psychological Association, 2001.
Nath Dwivedi, Kedar. *Post-Traumatic Stress Disorder in Children and Adolescents.* Northampton, UK: Whurr Publishers, Ltd., 2000.
Wilson, John P., Matthew J. Friedman, and Jacob D. Lindy. *Treating Psychological Trauma and PTSD.* New York: Guilford Publications, 2004.

■ PSYCHOLOGICAL ABUSE

Behavior that negatively impacts another person's emotional or psychological well-being. As with other forms of abuse, the goal of psychological abuse is to control the actions or feelings of the victim. Psychological abuse is also known as emotional abuse because it inflicts emotional, rather than physical, harm. Much of the behavior that makes up psychological abuse is verbal. Even though psychological abuse does not result in bodily damage or pain, studies suggest that it can have a negative effect on both one's mental and physical health.

WHAT CONSTITUTES PSYCHOLOGICAL ABUSE?

Although psychologists generally agree on the types of behaviors that qualify as physical abuse, they differ to some extent in their definitions of psychological abuse. According to a 1996 article in the *Journal of Emotional Abuse* titled "Defining Psychological Maltreatment in Domestic Violence Perpetrator Treatment Programs: Multiple Perspectives," some psychologists draw a distinction between emotional and psychological abuse. For example, some researchers define emotional abuse as actions that cause psychological pain or discomfort but do not necessarily imply a physical threat. They cite examples such as name-calling, yelling, or making false accusations. Psychological abuse, on the other hand, carries a threat of physical violence, either spoken or unspoken.

The test most widely used to identify psychological abuse is the Conflict Tactics Scale. It measures a range of abusive actions including passive behaviors (such as sulking or withdrawing from contact), hostile acts (such as insulting or swearing at a partner), threats, and physical violence. The Conflict Tactics Scale was the first attempt to classify a range of emotionally abusive behaviors. However, in recent years it has been criticized for not including many behaviors now commonly defined as psychological abuse.

The human rights watch group Amnesty International has developed its own definition of psychological violence. The definition closely reflects the ways that male **batterers** control and intimidate their partners. It includes the following behaviors:

- Isolating the victim from social contact
- Forcing the victim to work to exhaustion
- Exhibiting extreme possessiveness and jealousy
- Trying to convince the victim that he or she is insane or only imagines that the abuse took place
- Threatening to kill the partner or the partner's family or friends
- Threatening to commit suicide
- Degrading the victim through name-calling and humiliation
- Forcing the victim to take drugs or alcohol
- Offering promises, gifts, or actions that falsely suggest that the abuse will stop

The first test specifically designed to measure psychological abuse by male batterers is the Psychological Violence Toward Women Inventory. The developer of the test, psychologist Richard Tolman, studied the answers provided by both male batterers and **battered** females to 58 separate statements. He found that the responses fell into two categories of abusive behavior: domination/isolation and emotional/verbal. The former category included behaviors such as socially isolating the victim, demanding that the victim obey the abuser without question, and strictly enforcing traditional sex roles. The latter category involved behaviors such as insults, threats, withholding emotional support, and actions that degrade or demean the partner.

Perhaps the broadest definition of psychological abuse is the Duluth Model, developed by the Domestic Containment Program in Duluth, Minnesota. The program looks at battering from a social and political perspective rather than a psychological one. That is, it views the main source of abuse as the attitudes and values promoted by society rather than the psychological maladjustment of individuals. In an age in which physical strength is no longer necessary for survival, the program argues that abuse serves as a way for men to control the balance of power between the sexes. The list of behaviors considered psychological abuse by the Duluth Model is more comprehensive than other models and includes the use of:

- Threats or coercion
- Money or finances to control a victim
- "Male privilege" (treating a partner as a servant, making all decisions, and enforcing traditional sex roles)
- Children to manipulate a partner (threatening to take away the children or making the victim feel guilty about the way she raises the children)
- Behaviors that minimize the extent of the abuse or denials that it took place
- Claims that the victim is to blame for his or her abuse or that the victim's actions provoked the abusive behavior
- Social isolation to control the victim
- Monitors to watch where the victim goes or who the victim visits or talks to
- Jealousy to justify abusive behavior
- Verbal abuse including name-calling, yelling, insults, and degrading comments
- Intimidation (violent gestures, destroying property, abusing pets, or displaying a weapon)

There are few laws that relate to psychological or emotional abuse. In general, any threat of harm to a person is considered assault. Assault can be a purely verbal act, but most cases of assault involve some physical gesture, such as waving a fist at someone. If the assault involves a threat to kill the victim, it is considered aggravated assault. Stalking, defined as making unwanted contact with someone in a way that communicates a threat or causes the other person to fear for his or her safety, is also illegal, but definitions of the actions that constitute stalking vary from state to state. They include such actions as unwanted personal, phone, mail, or e-mail contact, unwanted gifts, vandalism, and verbal or physical threats. However, many other behaviors commonly considered psychological abuse, such as insults and name-calling, are not illegal acts.

TEENS SPEAK

I Could Never Understand My Father

I was always a good kid, a solid student, and a pretty fair athlete, but no matter what I did I never seemed to please him. No grade was good enough, no athletic accomplishment was outstanding enough, and nothing I did to help out around the house was up to his standards. It hurt and it was really frustrating. Why didn't he ever make me feel like I was worthwhile?

I remember the first time I made my high school football team. I wasn't particularly big or strong, and my father told me I should try out for football because it would "make a man out of me." He had played football in school and I thought that if I was able to make the team he'd be really proud of me. It was really hard work trying to beat out kids who were much bigger and faster than me, but I eventually made the team as the second-string tight end. I was so excited, I couldn't wait to get home and tell my dad the good news.

At dinner that evening I told my dad I made the team, and his first reaction was "Are you starting?" I was kind of surprised because I was thrilled just to make the team; I didn't think I had any chance to be a starter. I told him that I was backing up the tight end who started last year, but that the coach told me I'd probably get a lot of playing time, anyway. My dad was furious. He started yelling at me and called me a loser. He said I didn't have the heart to be a starter and that I'd always be a "second-stringer." I was crushed.

The next day I told coach about my father's reaction. The coach said that I should talk to the school counselor, so I did. I also told her about all the other times my dad ignored my accomplishments or made me feel like I wasn't measuring up to his standards. She told me that my dad was trying to use my feelings against me. He was controlling my behavior and emotions by making me feel like I couldn't do anything right. She called it "emotional abuse" and suggested that I talk to my mom about getting some counseling for the family. She said that it was the only way to make my dad realize what he was doing and to make him change his behavior.

I am really glad that I spoke to the counselor. I now realize that the way my dad acts is not my fault or because of anything I did. I hope my dad agrees to go to counseling because, in spite of everything, I still love him and want to make him proud of me. And I want to be proud of him too.

INCIDENCE AND SYMPTOMS OF
PSYCHOLOGICAL ABUSE

Incidences of psychological abuse are difficult to calculate, because most statistics on domestic violence and child abuse focus on physical abuses that result in some type of legal action. However, victims of physical abuse have often suffered emotional and psychological abuse as well. One of the few scientific examinations into this matter is the National Violence Against Women Survey reported in 2002 in the *American Journal of Preventive Medicine*. The survey included telephone interviews with over 16,000 adults in the United States. The questioners sought information about the participants' health status and history of abuse by a domestic partner.

The study found that 29 percent of the women surveyed, and 23 percent of the men, reported being victims of psychological, sexual, or physical abuse by a partner. Almost half of the female respondents who had suffered abuse experienced psychological abuse. More than three-quarters of the abused men had also been victims of psychological abuse.

Since psychological abuse leaves no outward marks, it may be difficult to detect. However, the following behaviors are considered warning signs:

- Low self-esteem
- Withdrawal, fearfulness, or **depression**
- Aggression or emotional instability
- Sleep disturbances
- Physical complaints with no medical basis
- Inappropriate behavior for age or development
- Extreme passiveness or dependency
- Attempted suicide or talk of suicide
- Expressions of shame, guilt, self-blame, or self-criticism

- Frequent crying
- Discomfort or nervousness around caregivers or relatives
- Avoidance of eye contact

EFFECTS OF PSYCHOLOGICAL ABUSE

One of the most surprising findings of the National Violence Against Women Survey was that physical and psychological abuse seem to have similar effects on victims. In the study, victims who reported suffering psychological abuse were also likely to develop **chronic** (long-term) physical or mental illnesses than victims who did not experience psychological abuse. Victims of psychological abuse were also more likely to report poor general health, **depression**, injuries, and drug and alcohol abuse. However, according to the study, verbal abuse did not have as strong a negative impact as other types of psychological abuse such as social isolation or financial control.

It would seem logical that a person suffering both physical and psychological abuse would be more likely to leave an abusive relationship than someone subjected to physical abuse alone. However, a 1999 study in the journal *Violence and Victims* titled "Psychological Abuse: Implications for Adjustment and Commitment to Leave Violent Partners" suggests that just the opposite may be true. The study asked 68 women living in emergency women's shelters to report on their experiences of physical and psychological abuse, how they coped with the abuse, their current psychological well-being, and the presence of any symptoms of post-traumatic stress disorder, or PTSD. PTSD is a severe psychological reaction to a stressful event that can include recurrent flashbacks of the event, nightmares, irritability, anxiety, fatigue, forgetfulness, and social withdrawal.

Fact Or Fiction?

Psychological abuse has a greater negative effect on children than it does on adults.

Fact: According to a 1996 article in the *Journal of Emotional Abuse* titled "Defining Psychological Maltreatment in Domestic Violence Perpetrator Treatment Programs: Multiple Perspectives," psychological abuse can be much more devastating for a young child than for an adolescent. The study reported that early emotional abuse can have profound, long-lasting effects similar to those experienced by victims of sexual or physical abuse. It also found that children of all ages seem to suffer more adverse effects from psychological abuse than do adults.

According to the study, victims who experienced both physical and psychological abuse displayed higher levels of PTSD than those who suffered physical abuse alone. Victims with lower levels of PTSD were more likely to express a desire to leave the abusive relationship. Those who had higher levels of PTSD showed less determination to leave. In addition, the study found that women who used emotion-based forms of coping with the abuse were more likely to have symptoms of PTSD than those who used a problem-focused coping mechanism. Examples of emotion-based coping include denying that the abuse occurred or trying to minimize its importance. Problem-focused coping techniques include confronting the abuser about the behavior or talking to a counselor about the abuse.

These studies clearly indicate that psychological abuse can be just as damaging to its victims as physical and sexual abuse. The fact that psychological abuse is so much more common than physical and sexual abuse suggests that serious attention needs to be paid to minimizing the potential for such abuse. However, there are no legal remedies for most forms of psychological abuse. Most treatment and counseling programs that address the issues of domestic partner abuse, child abuse, or elder abuse focus on treating victims of physical and emotional abuse. The recognition that victims of abuse often suffer from PTSD has raised awareness of the importance of addressing emotional and psychological aspects of abusive relationships. It is hoped that this greater awareness will help contribute to more effective efforts to reduce the incidence and effects of psychological abuse.

See also: Child Abuse; Domestic Partner Abuse; Elder Abuse; Legal Intervention; Post-traumatic Stress Disorder and Abuse; Rehabilitation and Treatment; Stalking; Women and Abuse

FURTHER READING
Jantz, Gregory L., and Ann McMurray. *Healing the Scars of Emotional Abuse.* Grand Rapids, MI: Fleming H. Revell Company, 2003.

O'Hagnn, Kieran. *Emotional and Psychological Abuse of Children.*
Maidenhead, UK: Open University Press, 1992.
Tamm Loring, Marti. *Emotional Abuse: The Trauma and the
Treatment.* San Francisco, CA: Jossey-Bass, 1998.

■ REHABILITATION AND TREATMENT

Actions taken to help victims recover from the trauma of abuse and to
change the behavior of perpetrators. Abuse can take a terrible physical and psychological toll on its victims. Victims often require emotional and material support to deal with the consequences of abuse.
Such support may include counseling, emergency housing, financial
support, and legal assistance. While helping victims is vital, treatment
alone is not a sufficient response to abuse. In order to end abuse, perpetrators need rehabilitation—help in overcoming patterns of abusive
behavior and learning healthier ways to interact with others.

TREATING ABUSE

A wide variety of institutions and individuals play a role in treating
victims of abuse. These include emergency hotlines, physicians and
medical personnel, counselors and psychiatrists, and support groups.
Even though these groups approach treatment from slightly different
perspectives, each makes a unique and valuable contribution.

Emergency help

Many states and communities sponsor emergency hotlines that can
offer support and advice for victims of abuse. In addition, the
National Domestic Violence Hotline (NDVH) connects people in all 50
states, Washington, D.C., Puerto Rico, and the U.S. Virgin Islands with
victim's services toll-free, 24 hours a day, 365 days a year. The NDVH
has a database of more than 4,000 shelters and service providers and
offers up-to-date information on domestic partner violence, local
shelters for **battered** women, legal advice, assistance programs, and
social service programs. People who are being abused by same-sex
partners can also call for advice and help.

Hotline services include:

■ Crisis intervention to help callers identify problems and
possible solutions, including making safety plans if
there is an emergency

- Information about resources on domestic violence, child abuse, sexual assault, intervention programs for batterers and victims, and criminal justice issues
- Referrals to shelters, social service agencies, legal services, and other helping organizations

Most communities also have emergency shelters or safe places where victims who fear for their safety can go to escape their abusers. Some of these facilities are operated by state or local government agencies such as Child Protective Services, while others are privately owned. In addition to a safe place to stay, many shelters also offer victims medical and legal help and psychological counseling.

Medical treatment

Many victims of abuse require immediate medical treatment for their injuries. In 1999 the Department of Justice reported that 37 percent of all women who sought care in hospital emergency rooms for violence-related injuries were injured by a current or former spouse, boyfriend, or girlfriend. According to a 1992 article in the magazine *American Medical News* titled "The Billion Dollar Epidemic," a study at Rush Medical Center in Chicago found that the average charge for medical service provided to abused women, children, and older adults is $1,633 per person. This works out to a annual total of over $857 million nationwide.

A 1999 study published in the *Journal of Family Practice* found that victims of domestic violence cost the health care system much more than other patients. According to "Intimate Partner Violence against Women: Do Victims Cost Health Plans More?" health-care providers spent an average of $1,755 more per year on victims of domestic and child abuse than on their other patients. The study urged physicians to make efforts to identify family violence early to reduce the damage to victims and the costs to the health-care industry.

Despite the high incidence of domestic abuse in the United States, family physicians have been slow to recognize the problem. According to a study published by the *Journal of the American Medical Association* in 1999, fewer than 10 percent of primary care physicians routinely screen patients for domestic violence during regular office visits. The American Medical Association (AMA) also reported that hospital emergency departments only identify about 5 percent of abuse cases.

The AMA and other medical groups are working to train emergency room personnel, family doctors, and nurses to screen patients for abuse. This includes identifying injuries common to family abuse, such as:

- Injuries around the face, head, and neck
- Painful, tender, or swollen abdomen or genitals
- Internal injuries or bleeding
- Cracked or broken bones
- Burns, bruises, or healed scars

Medical professionals also are becoming more sensitive to behavioral indicators of abuse such as:

- **Depression**
- Suicidal thoughts
- Drug or alcohol use
- Anxiety or nervousness
- Shame or embarrassment
- Being accompanied by a partner who will not leave and answers all questions
- Jealousy and possessiveness by the partner

Medical personnel who suspect abuse are encouraged to ask the patient if they are being victimized. Many victims who are afraid for their safety will deny that abuse is occurring, especially if the abuser is present. Physicians and nurses try to interview patients in private if possible and offer them a safe place to stay if they report the abuse. Medical personnel also try to educate the victim about the danger of continued abuse. They advise victims of the importance of making a safety plan to escape if the abuse becomes serious. Victims are reassured that the abuse is not their fault and reminded that there are agencies that can assist them.

It can be particularly difficult to obtain information about abuse from a child. He or she may be too ashamed or embarrassed to discuss the abuse, or fear retaliation from the abuser. Young children who have been abused may not be able to understand the incident or communicate to an adult what happened. For these reasons medical personnel must be especially alert to physical or behavioral signs of abuse in children.

Support groups

Victims of abuse need the opportunity to connect with other people and talk about their experiences. For many victims, **support groups** are an important resource. They offer an environment in which victims can admit and discuss their abuse without fear of ridicule or embarrassment because all of the members have gone through the same experience. Support groups are made up of people who are at various stages of recovery from the abuse they experienced. Survivors who have begun to change their lives can be role models for those who are just starting to recover from abuse. The survivors are proof that people can recover and lead healthy lives. Many groups have a facilitator to guide the group's discussions and help the members benefit each other.

Like emergency shelters, support groups are set up and run by a variety of organizations. Some are associated with churches or religious groups, while others are run by local mental health associations. Many are sponsored by local family shelters or shelters for battered women, and others are independently organized by individuals who have themselves suffered abuse and wish to help other abuse victims. Larger communities may have support groups for specific populations of battered women, such as lesbians or women of color. In smaller communities, groups for battered women include women of all population groups. Most support groups for victims of partner abuse are for women only so that the women will feel safe and express themselves freely. Groups for battered men are less common, except in larger communities with active gay men's organizations. However, these groups rarely address the needs of heterosexual men abused by female partners.

TEENS SPEAK

After I Broke Up with My Boyfriend I Was Afraid to Date Again

I didn't think I could make good decisions about guys and didn't want to take another chance of ending up with a jerk. Not that I called it abuse when it was happening. I denied it because I didn't know that I deserved better. Then a friend told me about a support group at school. It was called something like "Women's Empowerment." Maybe on some level I did know I had been a victim, because I thought, "I need to learn to stand up for myself."

After I joined the group, I realized that it was about abuse and that I wasn't the only one who experienced it. We had a group leader, who encouraged us to talk to one another, even outside of the group. (Of course, she kept reminding us not to talk to outsiders about what other group members said.)

The group leader said that we were our own best teachers, but she also taught us about patterns of abuse and staying safe. Most importantly, she taught us skills like assertiveness, knowing what we feel, expressing our feelings, and even how to disagree and settle conflicts.

I think it was a good group, and the girls I was in the group with are now my friends for life. I'm not dating anyone right now, not because I am afraid to, but because I don't need a guy in my life for me to feel good about myself. I realized from group that I had been willing to settle for any guy, just to have someone. But I deserve better than that.

REHABILITATION

Treatment addresses the immediate physical and emotional needs of abuse victims, but rehabilitation is the key to long-term healing of the wounds of abuse. In rehabilitation, victims address the causes of abuse and work to change behavior patterns that may lead to abuse. These efforts include counseling and therapy aimed at both the victims and the perpetrators of abuse.

Counseling for domestic abuse

The most common type of therapy (psychological treatment) for couples trying to overcome domestic abuse is called gender-specific treatment (GST). In GST, victims and perpetrators of abuse meet in same-sex groups to discuss issues related to the abuse. Those who practice this theory hold abusers responsible for their aggressive behavior. The goal is to encourage them to change their controlling and violent behavior.

An alternative approach to GST is called conjoint treatment, or couples therapy. In conjoint treatment, the couple meets with a counselor to discuss issues relating to abuse. Conjoint therapy is based on the belief that the personal interaction between partners plays a major role in domestic violence. Therefore, therapists focus on improving communication between partners rather than changing the behavior of one partner. Opponents of conjoint therapy argue that it can be dangerous to treat the victim and perpetrator together. They fear that the discussion may lead to violence after the counseling session is over. However, those who prefer conjoint therapy claim that GST does not promote communication between the abuser and the victim, which they feel is essential for change.

A comparison of the two therapies shows that both have similar rates of effectiveness in reducing marital violence. A 1999 study titled "Treatment of Wife Abuse: A Comparison of Gender-Specific and Conjoint Approaches" found no significant differences in effectiveness between the two. In both forms of therapy about 39 percent of abusive husbands completely stopped physical aggression during treatment. In the year prior to treatment, 73 percent of husbands in the study severely abused their wives; this number fell to 34 percent in the year following treatment.

Despite encouraging short-term reductions in violence, neither therapy resulted in significant long-term changes in behavior. According to the study, 75 percent of the husbands who received therapy used some form of physical aggression against their wives in the year following treatment. And over a third continued to severely abuse their wives in the following year. In addition, 47 percent of the couples dropped out of therapy before completing the program. Most counseling programs for batterers have a similar dropout rate, which is a serious drawback to many domestic violence treatment programs.

Other programs that treat domestic abusers use a variety of techniques. For example, the University of Massachusetts Memorial Medical Center offers domestic violence treatment programs that focus on anger management. The program director, Dr. Lynn Dowd, says that most participants have trouble finding appropriate ways to express anger. The program uses videos, discussions, and other exercises to help participants understand how they react to stressful situations and find nonviolent responses to those situations. Another program, based at Rhode Island Hospital, teaches participants about the biology of anger. It helps abusers recognize the physical signs of anger and teaches them relaxation techniques to calm themselves whenever they feel angry. As promising as some of these programs are, counselors who treat batterers say that there are still far too few programs in the United States.

Fact Or Fiction?

Batterers can learn to control their abusive behavior.

Fact: According to a 2000 article in the *Journal of Interpersonal Violence*, former batterers were able to successfully change their behavior using certain strategies. "Change among Batterers: Examining Men's Success Stories" found four factors that were important in helping abusive men change their behavior:

1. Recognizing and taking responsibility for their abusive behavior

2. Developing empathy for others, especially their partners

3. Recognizing that their partners are individuals who have a right to their own feelings

4. Improving skills for communication needs and feelings, including anger management, conflict resolution, learning how to listen, and learning how to share intimate feelings

Counseling for child abuse

Most counseling programs for abused children have focused on treating the effects of child sexual abuse. According to a 2001 article "Treatment Outcome Research: How Effective are Treatments for Abused Children?" group treatment was more effective than individual treatment in raising victims' self-esteem but had little effect on anxiety or depression. In addition, cognitive-behavioral therapy (CBT) was found to be more effective than standard counseling or psychotherapy. CBT involves teaching the abused child to change the way he or she thinks about the abuse in order to relieve some of the negative emotions surrounding abuse. For example, many children blame themselves for the abuse. CBT teaches them that they are not to blame and helps them understand and deal with their emotions.

The same article pointed out that far fewer studies have focused on treatment of the physical abuse of children. In its 2002 publication

World Report on Violence and Health, the World Health Organization offers an example of a peer treatment program for physically abused children. The program brings together abused preschool children who are socially withdrawn with children who have better social skills. Those children are taught to act as role models for the children who are more withdrawn. They model such behaviors as offering toys to the withdrawn children. Such therapy has proven to be effective in helping withdrawn victims of abuse improve their social interaction with peers. However, aggressive children showed increased negative behavior with peer therapy groups. They had better results with CBT, leading to improvements in child behavior and reductions in distress, child-to-parent violence, and family conflict.

Treatments for **neglect** of children have also been studied less thoroughly. Most interventions for neglect focus on treating the **caregiver** but not the child. Traditional counseling has had little effect in helping children overcome the trauma of neglect. An approach that combines behavioral changes with social support and active intervention by social agencies seems to offer the best hope for victims of neglect.

In recent years therapists have turned their attention to children who witness domestic violence. According to Alicia Lieberman, a child development specialist and professor of psychiatry at the University of California at San Francisco, witnessing domestic violence may increase a child's risk of becoming an abusive adult. Lieberman conducted a study in which 45 pairs of abused mothers and children were visited by a therapist every week for a year. The therapists helped the mothers and children resolve conflicts that might damage their relationship. The study found that only two of the children developed the symptoms of extreme anxiety that abused children typically show. Such studies hold out hope that children who witness domestic violence can overcome the emotional and psychological scars of that experience and break the cycle of abuse as adults.

Q & A

Question: Are there school programs for teen boys who want to be sure they don't become abusers?

Answer: Some schools or youth programs teach about relationships and relationship violence. However, the programs are not common enough given the frequency of teen dating violence. There may be special programs through a local domestic violence shelter, mental health department, or other mental health agency. Many school health classes also cover relationship issues. Colleges may offer their students special workshops. The goal of these programs is to help students understand that they have choices. Using violence is a choice, even though it is a poor choice. No one can make you hit someone. These programs also look at male stereotypes and explain why males should reject those negative images.

COMMUNITY AND FAMILY RESPONSES

Family members and members of the wider community also have a part to play in helping victims overcome abuse. In 1994, the American Medical Association brought together a wide range of people to discuss the ways in which communities can reduce family violence and its effects. One recommendation was the creation of local family violence councils that include medical personnel, lawyers, clergy, therapists, educators, substance abuse counselors, corrections officials, representatives from shelters and other community agencies, rehabilitated offenders, survivors of abuse, and other concerned citizens.

The goals of these councils and similar community initiatives include:

- Improving coordination and communication among hospitals, social service agencies, and law enforcement

- Providing training opportunities for those who treat and counsel abuse victims

- Sharing intervention strategies

- Improving the response of law enforcement and the courts to instances of abuse

- Developing policies and procedures for providing services to victims of abuse

- Ensuring that services are not duplicated and that there are the necessary services in place for abuse survivors, their families, and the abusers

- Ensuring that effective prevention and treatment programs are available

- Promoting and presenting educational programs in schools

Families in which abuse occurs need to learn new interpersonal and coping skills so that future generations do not resort to violence. Organizations such as Parents Anonymous can help them accomplish this goal. Parents Anonymous is the oldest national child abuse prevention organization in the country. It is dedicated to strengthening families and has community-based chapters around the country. Parents who are abusive or have a tendency to exhibit violent behavior go to learn personal and interpersonal skills that help them handle the stresses that can lead to anger and violent behavior. By learning and modeling these new skills, they also teach their children that violence is not the solution to problems. In this way they can break the cycle of violence.

Organizations such as Parents Anonymous and other support and counseling groups teach such valuable skills as:

- Self-control. By learning to identify and express feelings, parents and partners use meaningful words instead of physical or verbal violence to express anger or frustration. It is amazing how much better it feels just to be able to put a name to a feeling and let others know how you feel. This is the first step toward talking out the problem, exploring options, or asking for what you need.

- Communication skills. People are not mind readers. They can only guess at what another person wants. Sometimes they guess wrong or don't guess at all, and the other person gets angry and frustrated. People in treatment for violent behavior need to learn to ask for what they want or need and not expect their partner or children automatically to know. Better communication skills lead to self-control.

- Negotiation. Negotiation is the skill of being able to "give and take," compromise, and cooperate. It is a skill necessary in any close relationship so that both parties can participate fully in making decisions and feel that they have been heard. No one can get his or her way all the time, but by learning to negotiate, two people can work out a win-win solution to a disagreement.

- Mediation. When two people can't work out a compromise or agreement through direct negotiation, they may need help from another person. That person can be an objective mediator. The mediator can help two people reach a solution they both can live with, even if neither one is completely happy with the outcome.

Increasing the quality of communication allows family members to honestly explore issues that can lead to conflict and possibly violence. By contrast, failure to effectively communicate leads to secrecy and denial, which can help perpetuate abuse that might occur. Healthy family dynamics are an essential part of preventing as well as dealing with abuse and domestic violence.

See also: Abusers, Common Traits of; Child Abuse; Child Sexual Abuse; Domestic Partner Abuse; Men and Abuse; Sexual Abuse; Sexual Assault; Women and Abuse

FURTHER READING
Campbell, Jacquelyn C. *Empowering Survivors of Abuse: Health Care, Battered Women and Their Children.* Thousand Oaks, CA: Sage Publications, 1998.
Dobash, R. Emerson, Russell P. Dobash, Kate Cavanagh, et al. *Changing Violent Men.* Thousand Oaks, CA: Sage Publications, 1999.
Lee, Mo Yee, John Sebold, and Adriana Uken. *Solution-Focused Treatment of Domestic Violence Offenders: Accountability for Change.* New York: Oxford University Press, 2003.
Mills, Linda. *Insult to Injury: Rethinking Our Responses to Intimate Abuse.* Princeton, NJ: Princeton University Press, 2003.
Salter, Anna C. *Transforming Trauma: A Guide to Understanding and Treating Adult Survivors of Child Sexual Abuse.* Thousand Oaks, CA: Sage Publications, 1995.
Wiehe, Vernon R. *Understanding Family Violence: Treating and Preventing Partner, Child, Sibling, and Elder Abuse.* Thousand Oaks, CA: Sage Publications, 1998.

■ SELF-MUTILATION
Deliberately harming oneself without the intent to commit suicide is called self-mutilation (also known as self-injury or self-harm). Self-mutilation is a complex group of behaviors that have a variety of causes. Research has linked self-mutilation to emotional and psychological shocks such as child abuse and **neglect**, as well as to biological differences in the brain chemistry of those who self-mutilate.

TYPES OF SELF-MUTILATION

In his 1996 book *Bodies under Siege: Self-Mutilation and Body Modification in Culture and Psychiatry*," psychiatrist A.R. Favazza of the Johns Hopkins University Medical Center classifies instances of self-mutilation as major, stereotypic, or superficial. Major self-mutilation, which involves serious injury such as amputating a limb or gouging out an eye, is very rare and usually practiced by people suffering from serious psychological disorders. Stereotypic self-mutilation refers to the kind of repeated and automatic behaviors such as head-banging seen in autistic or mentally retarded individuals. Superficial self-mutilation is the most common type. It includes cutting, burning, scratching, failing to let wounds heal, and even breaking bones. Because most of these self-inflicted injuries are cuts, self-mutilation is commonly referred to as "cutting."

Within the category of superficial self-mutilation, Favazza identifies three types of injury. Compulsive injuries include acts such as hair-pulling and skin-picking that are often performed as part of a ritual. Compulsive self-mutilation is associated with the psychological condition known as obsessive-compulsive disorder, in which a person performs certain actions repeatedly in exactly the same way, usually as a way to reduce tension or anxiety.

Episodic self-harm occurs when people who don't think of themselves as self-mutilators occasionally strike out at themselves. Although this type of self-mutilation is not ongoing, it is usually a sign of an underlying psychological disorder. Episodic self-harm can, however, turn into a recurring pattern of behavior. The person begins to think more often about self-mutilation and to identify himself or herself as a self-mutilator. Psychiatrists suggest that this type of behavior arises from stressful situations and eventually becomes an automatic response to the stress. It has been compared to a nicotine addict reaching for a cigarette to cope with stressful circumstances.

Fact Or Fiction?

Self-mutilation is an attempt to commit suicide.

Fact: Self-mutilation is a way of coping with living, not a way of dying. It is intended to release pain, often to keep from killing oneself. In contrast to self-mutilation, attempted suicide does not provide relief from stress, is not repeated as frequently, and is not intended to communicate unspoken emotional states. People who practice self-mutilation may attempt suicide out of desperation, but the goal of self-mutilation itself is not to take one's own life.

CHARACTERISTICS OF SELF-MUTILATORS

Research into self-mutilation has revealed a general picture of those who harm themselves. Such individuals suffer from a variety of emotional and psychological problems, including:

- Self-hatred
- Extreme sensitivity to rejection
- Chronic (long-term) anger, particularly at themselves
- Aggressiveness
- Inability to control impulses
- Inability to plan for the future
- **Depression**
- Anxiety
- Irritability
- Poor coping skills

A 1992 study in the *American Journal of Psychiatry*, "Self-mutilation in Personality Disorders: Psychological and Biological Correlates," found that self-mutilators had long-standing problems with anger and anxiety. The 1993 book *Cognitive-Behavioral Treatment of Borderline Personality Disorder* reported that most self-mutilators act only on their immediate feelings and impulses and rarely consider the long-term consequences of their actions.

According to a 1998 article in the journal *Suicide and Life Threatening Behavior* titled "Self-mutilation and Eating Disorders," about 750 of every 100,000 Americans (three-quarters of 1 percent) are self-mutilators. In the study, 97 percent of those who admitted to self-harm were female. The article reported that the "typical" self-mutilator is an intelligent, well-educated, middle-class woman in her mid-20s to early 30s. The average respondent in the study had been inflicting self-harm since her teens, had a history of physical or sexual abuse, and had at least one alcoholic parent. Many of the young women surveyed also had eating disorders. Other studies have confirmed that women are more likely to self-mutilate than men but found smaller sex differences. E-mail from online surveys and support sites suggest that females comprise 67–85 percent of all cases of self-mutilation.

CAUSES OF SELF-MUTILATION

Most people find self-mutilation puzzling and disturbing. They tend to consider such behavior senseless or irrational. However, researchers suggest that self-mutilation meets certain emotional or psychological needs. A large number of studies have identified various motivations for self-mutilation. They can be grouped into three general categories: affect regulation, communication, and control/punishment.

Affect regulation is an attempt to restore one's emotional or psychological balance after experiencing a stressful event or disturbing feelings. According to this explanation, self-mutilation provides relief from intense feelings with which a person is unable to cope. A 1995 study in the *Journal of Abnormal Psychology* titled "The Psychophysiology of Self-mutilation" argues that self-injury is an effective way for some people to relieve emotional or psychological tension.

Another theory suggests that self-mutilation is a way for certain individuals to communicate feelings they cannot put into words. A 1996 article in the journal *Comprehensive Psychiatry* titled "The Relationship between Dissociative Symptoms, Alexithymia, Impulsivity, Sexual Abuse, and Self-mutilation," found that self-mutilators often cannot describe or name the emotions they feel before they hurt themselves. Instead of verbalizing their feelings, they try to communicate them through self-mutilation.

The 1994 book *Women Who Hurt Themselves: A Book of Hope and Understanding* tries to explain why so many self-mutilators are women. According to the author, female self-mutilation stems from the fact that girls are taught to repress violent urges or behaviors. Instead of striking out at others when they feel rage, they turn their anger inward through acts of self-mutilation. A related theory was put forward in *Cognitive-Behavioral Treatment of Borderline Personality Disorder.* This theory states that self-mutilation comes from repeatedly being told that one's feelings are wrong, inappropriate, or invalid. The book suggests that male self-mutilation stems from the fact that men are raised to hold in their emotions rather than express them freely. A man who feels it is inappropriate to express certain emotions verbally may instead act them out through self-mutilation.

A third general theory is based on the idea that self-mutilation is a way to gain a sense of control over stressful situations or their own impulses. A 1995 article "The Significance of Aggression and Impulsivity for Self-mutilative Behavior" suggests that self-mutilators disapprove of their aggressive feelings and use self-harm as a way to suppress them. In effect, they harm themselves to control their feelings of aggression toward others. The study found that people who harm themselves experience strong psychological relief after an episode of self-mutilation even though they have negative feelings afterward.

According to a 1991 article in the *American Journal of Psychiatry* titled "Childhood Origins of Self-destructive Behavior," physical and sexual abuse, **neglect**, and a disruptive family environment in childhood and adolescence are related to both the frequency and the seriousness of self-mutilation. The earlier one suffers abuse, the more likely one is to inflict self-harm and the more damage one does. Childhood neglect was found to be the best predictor of later self-mutilation. These results are supported by a 1989 study reported in the *American Journal of Psychiatry* in which women began to engage in self-mutilation after becoming victims of traumatic rape.

Several studies have linked self-mutilation to reduced levels of the **neurotransmitter** serotonin. Neurotransmitters are chemicals that allow nerve cells to communicate with one another to maintain normal physical and psychological functioning. Changes in the amount of neurotransmitters available for use by nerve cells can produce profound changes in behavior. Reduced levels of serotonin have been linked to increased aggression and depression. In a 1994 article "Long-term Consequences of Childhood Physical Abuse," the journal *Psychological Bulletin* suggests that reduced levels of serotonin may explain the connection between childhood abuse and self-mutilation.

TEENS SPEAK

Whenever I Cut Myself, I Feel Better

I don't know how to describe it. Sometimes it just feels like I have released a pressure valve and the steam comes out. I think the first time I did it was when I was about 14. Then I started cutting for just about anything that made me feel bad. I don't think that I was really depressed, but I did feel down a lot and I didn't feel very good about myself. I never felt that I mattered to anyone.

At first I used a razor and then a knife. Somehow, seeing my own blood was a way to prove I was alive. I cut my arms and legs and I wore baggy clothes so no one could see the scars. It wasn't that I wanted to die or anything. It was just a way to feel better. I don't remember it ever hurting physically. The cutting was like a painkiller for my emotions. I did it whenever I needed to, first every few weeks, then once a week, and then a few times a day! I felt driven to hurt myself, like it was an addiction. I also burned myself with matches and cigarettes.

My mother started to notice scars and I finally told her the truth. I think admitting it helped me stop. I was ashamed, but she got me help. The therapist told me to draw on my arms with a red pen or to hold ice if I felt like hurting myself. It was hard to stop cutting. It's been four years since I cut myself, but I still think about it and am tempted when I feel bad. I am now better at talking about my feelings and writing in my journal.

TREATING SELF-MUTILATION

Researchers have suggested several different strategies for treating self-mutilation, including psychological and biological approaches to therapy. One approach favored by many professionals is rational-emotive therapy (RET), developed by psychologist Albert Ellis. Self-mutilators tend to allow their current feelings and emotions to determine their thoughts and actions, but RET is based on the idea that your thoughts control your feelings, not vice versa.

Rational-emotive therapy argues that negative emotions are the result of years of thinking and responding to situations in a particular way. RET attempts to help patients learn to control negative emotions by teaching them to rethink their reactions to stressful situations. For example, suppose a close friend or intimate partner forgets to call when promised. Someone who lets emotions control his or her thoughts may automatically assume that the other person deliberately chose not to call. The person expecting the call feels rejected, and he or she may deal with those feelings by engaging in self-mutilation. Using RET, a therapist may encourage the person to interpret the situation differently. The patient is asked to consider other explanations for the failure to call. For example, the other person may have been too busy to call or their cell phone may have run out of power.

Q & A

Question: What can I do to help a friend who is hurting himself or herself?

Answer: There are several actions you should take if you know someone who is inflicting self-harm, including:

- Talking to your friend about self-mutilation. This can help remove the secrecy and shame that surrounds self-inflicted injury and encourage the person to seek professional help.
- Ask how you can be supportive and what you can do to help
- Spend time with your friend so he or she has less opportunity to inflict self-harm
- Do not discourage your friend from self-mutilation. He or she probably uses it to deal with stress and likely has no other coping mechanisms to rely on.
- Try to understand how severe the problem is and avoid negative judgments about your friend's behavior

Another approach to treatment is combining psychotherapy methods such as RET with drug treatment. Favazza recommends that self-mutilators take a drug that helps increase the amount of serotonin in the nervous system, thus addressing the underlying biological cause of the behavior and helping to get the self-mutilation under control relatively quickly. He then suggests following drug treatment with some form of psychotherapy, such as RET, to address the psychological causes of self-harm.

While the ultimate goal of therapy for self-mutilation is to stop self-destructive behavior, that is not necessarily a short-term priority. Because self-mutilation is often used as a way to cope with stress, trying to eliminate it too quickly may increase a patient's stress. In addition, many people who self-mutilate have no other mechanisms for coping with stress. One suggestion is for the therapist to tolerate self-mutilation but to let the patient know that such behavior has consequences. For example, the therapist might instruct the patient to contact him or her upon feeling the urge to self-mutilate but avoid contact for some time after any act of self-harm. The idea is to give the patient a chance to communicate his or her feelings without resorting to self-mutilation. Such an approach also lets the patient know that self-mutilation will have negative effects but that those effects are temporary.

See also: Abuse, Theories of; Child Abuse; Women and Abuse

FURTHER READING

Alderman, Tracy. *The Scarred Soul: Understanding and Ending Self-inflicted Violence.* Oakland, CA: New Harbinger Publications, 1997.

Levenkron, Steven. *Cutting: Understanding and Overcoming Self-mutilation.* New York: W. W. Norton & Company, 1999.

Strong, Marilee. *A Bright Red Scream: Self-mutilation and the Language of Pain.* New York: Penguin Books, 1999.

Turner, V. J. *Secret Scars: Uncovering and Understanding the Addiction of Self-injury.* Center City, MN: Hazelden Publishing and Educational Services, 2002.

Winkler, Kathleen. *Cutting and Self-mutilation: When Teens Injure Themselves.* Berkeley Heights, NJ: Enslow Publishers, 2003.

■ SEXUAL ABUSE

The use of sex to control the actions or behaviors of another person. Sexual abuse typically involves coercion or pressure rather than physical force or the threat of violence. The most common forms of sexual abuse are **sexual harassment** and **sexual exploitation**. Both sexual harassment and sexual exploitation involve similar behaviors. However, sexual harassment can occur between any two individuals, while sexual exploitation takes place between a more powerful perpetrator and a less powerful victim. Sexual abuse may or may not be illegal, depending upon the circumstances. However, regardless of whether or not a particular act is illegal, sexual abuse is psychologically harmful to its victims.

SEXUAL HARASSMENT

Sexual harassment involves persistent and unwelcome acts or comments of a sexual nature, including:

- Unwelcome sexual advances;
- Requests for sexual favors;
- Physical touching of a sexual nature; or
- Demeaning or degrading sexual comments.

There are two basic types of sexual harassment: quid pro quo and hostile environment. *Quid pro quo* is a Latin phrase meaning "this for that." In quid pro quo harassment, a person offers someone favors in return for sex or threatens some type of harm if the person refuses to have sex. For example, a boy offering to buy his girlfriend an expensive gift in exchange for having sex with him is an example of quid pro quo sexual harassment. A boy who threatens to break up with his girlfriend if she will not have sex with him is also committing quid pro quo sexual harassment. Quid pro quo harassment can happen in many different settings: at a party, in a school environment, and on the job.

By contrast, hostile environment harassment occurs in a specific setting, such as a school or workplace. A hostile environment exists when harassment is so frequent and intimidating that the victim feels threatened or is unable to enjoy the benefits of the environment. For example, a hostile environment exists at school if a student is unable to participate in or benefit from school activities because of sexual harassment by another student.

Sexual harassment at school

According to the U.S. Department of Education pamphlet "Sexual Harassment: It's Not Academic," sexual harassment is a serious problem at all levels of the educational system from elementary school to college. Title IX of the Education Amendments of 1972 prohibits sex discrimination—including sexual harassment—in public schools. The Department of Education claims that sexual harassment in school undermines efforts to create a safe and nondiscriminatory learning environment.

In the 2000 case *Vance v. Spencer County Public School District*, the U.S. Sixth Circuit Court of Appeals ruled that schools can be held liable in cases of student-on-student sexual harassment if school officials are aware of the harassment and do nothing to stop it. The case involved a student in a Kentucky school who claimed her classmates subjected her to physical and verbal abuse of a sexual nature over a period of three years. Despite verbal and written complaints by the girl's mother, school officials never disciplined the students involved, although they did speak with the harassers about their behavior. In 1995, the girl's mother filed a lawsuit against the school under Title IX. The jury in the case ruled against the school district and ordered the district to pay $220,000 in damages. The district appealed the decision, but the appeals court upheld the original verdict. That same year, the U.S. Supreme Court upheld a similar ruling in *Davis v. Monroe Board of Education*. The decision confirmed that schools bear the responsibility of stopping sexual harassment whenever they are aware that such behavior is occurring.

TEENS SPEAK

He Started by Making Sexual Comments about My Body or the Way I Dressed

When I moved to a new school last year I was a little nervous because I was leaving most of my friends but also kind of excited about making new ones. Now I wish I had never left my old school. None of the students in the new school was very friendly and pretty soon this boy named Eric started to hassle me.

Sometimes Eric called me "babe" and made these really nasty faces. I was really scared and didn't know what to do. He was a popular boy and I was just a new kid that nobody knew. When I tried to talk to other kids about it, they just laughed or said "that's the way Eric is." One girl even said I should be flattered because he only picked on girls he thought were cute. I thought about telling a teacher, but he hadn't touched me or hurt me in any way; he just made me uncomfortable.

Then one day, when I was at my locker between classes, I felt someone touching me from behind. I looked around and it was Eric. He started to touch me again and began laughing at me, saying how I really liked it and that I should just stop fighting him. I got away from him and ran straight to the assistant principal's office. I talked to the assistant principal and told her what happened. I also told her that I knew Eric was harassing other girls but they were too afraid to talk about it. I wasn't sure the assistant principal would do anything, but she told me that if Eric was bothering me she'd make sure he stopped.

I found out later that the assistant principal talked to some other students who told her Eric had bothered them too. The school suspended Eric, and since he came back from suspension he hasn't bothered me or anyone else. I realize now that silence only helps protect the harasser. I'm glad I decided to speak up, otherwise Eric might still be harassing other girls and me.

Sexual harassment at work
Research shows that workplace sexual harassment is a widespread problem. A 1994 poll by Lou Harris and Associates found that 31 percent of female workers reported they had been sexually harassed at their place of employment. In 70 percent of those cases the harasser was either the victim's supervisor or another senior-level employee, and all of the perpetrators were men. According to the poll, men also suffer sexual harassment at work but much less frequently than women. Only 7 percent of the men surveyed had been sexually harassed at the workplace. Most of them (59 percent) said the perpetrator was female.

Sexual harassment not only harms its victims but also has an adverse effect on the workplace. A 1990 survey in *Working Woman* magazine found that sexual harassment can cost large businesses millions of dollars each year in absenteeism, lost productivity, employee turnover, and legal costs associated with harassment lawsuits. In 2003, businesses involved in sexual harassment suits paid victims some $50 million in damages.

SEXUAL EXPLOITATION
Sexual exploitation occurs when a person uses a position of power or authority to coerce someone to have sex. It is similar to sexual harassment in that it involves unwanted sexual attention. However, sexual exploitation always involves a difference in power between the perpetrator and victim. The perpetrator uses this power to obtain sexual favors from the victim. An example of sexual exploitation would be a manager threatening to fire an employee who did not agree to have sex.

Sexual exploitation can also occur when dealing with professionals such as doctors, nurses, counselors, social workers, law enforcement officials, and lawyers. The specialized knowledge such individuals possess gives them significant power over people who seek their help. A doctor, for example, may literally hold the power of life and death over his or her patients. Some professionals use this power to coerce sex from their clients or patients. Because professional power can be abused, most helping professions have established codes of conduct that prohibit sexual relationships between members of those fields and their clients.

EFFECTS OF SEXUAL HARASSMENT AND EXPLOITATION

Sexual harassment can have devastating physical and psychological effects. According to the counseling center at the University of Oregon, psychological reactions to sexual harassment may include:

- **Depression**
- Anxiety, fear, shock, and denial
- Anger, frustration, and irritability
- Insecurity, embarrassment, and feelings of betrayal
- Confusion and feelings of powerlessness
- Shame, guilt, and self-blame
- Low self-esteem

Among physical symptoms caused by sexual harassment are:

- Headaches
- Tiredness, listlessness, or lack of energy
- Stomach and intestinal problems
- Skin reactions such as rashes or acne
- Weight changes
- Sleep disturbances and nightmares
- Panic reactions and phobias (irrational fears)
- Sexual problems

Sexual exploitation by professionals can result in many of the same psychological difficulties as sexual harassment. The American Psychological Association's *Diagnostic and Statistical Manual of Mental*

Disorders lists a number of possible consequences of sexual exploitation, including:

- Lowered self-esteem
- Depression and anxiety
- Post-traumatic stress disorder (PTSD)
- Nightmares and insomnia
- Relationship difficulties and divorce
- Substance abuse
- Increased risk of suicide

RESPONDING TO SEXUAL HARASSMENT AND EXPLOITATION

The proper response to sexual harassment depends upon the individuals involved and the setting in which it occurs. If the power between the parties is roughly equal, the victim should speak to the perpetrator. For example, the United States Equal Employment Opportunity Commission (EEOC) recommends that a victim of sexual harassment in the workplace tell the harasser that such behavior is unwelcome and demand that it stop.

However, in situations where the perpetrator holds physical, psychological, or financial power over the victim, harassment should be reported to an outside authority. For example, if a doctor is sexually exploiting a patient, the victim should contact the state medical board or other agency that licenses physicians. Some states now have laws that prohibit members of certain professions from having sexual relations with patients—even former patients. Similarly, the Department of Education recommends that students contact a school official immediately if they are being harassed by a teacher, staff member, or another student.

Q & A

Question: My stepbrother touches me in a way I am not comfortable with. What should I do?

Answer: Tell your stepbrother that you will not tolerate his touching you anymore. Tell him that you want his behavior to stop. If he does not stop, try talking to your parents. Parents are the people who need to know what is happening, but there are many reasons you may be reluctant to tell your parents about being abused, including:

- Fearing that parents will not believe you or will not do anything about it
- Fearing your stepbrother may hurt you if you do tell
- Uncertainty as to whether the behavior is sexual abuse or a misunderstanding of your stepbrother's actions
- Blaming yourself for the behavior

If you cannot tell your parents or they do nothing, call a local rape crisis center or rape hotline and talk about the problem with a trained counselor. You can also talk to other adults in your life. Some adults, such as teachers and counselors, are legally required to report such abuse to law enforcement authorities or agencies such as Child Protective Services.

Of course, the best way to deal with sexual harassment or exploitation is to prevent it from happening. The Department of Education's Office for Civil Rights has issued guidelines to help prevent sexual harassment at school. Their suggestions include:

- Developing a school policy that defines sexual harassment and states clearly that it will not be tolerated
- Establishing a procedure for filing complaints of sexual harassment
- Conducting periodic staff training in identifying and dealing with sexual harassment
- Conducting periodic sexual harassment awareness classes for students
- Establishing discussion groups where students can talk about sexual harassment and how to respond to it
- Working with students and teachers to develop effective ways to deal with sexual harassment

Similar steps can be taken to prevent sexual harassment in the workplace. The EEOC suggests that management make all employees aware that it will not tolerate sexual harassment. Businesses should provide all employees with a copy of the company policy regarding sexual harassment as well as procedures for filing complaints. If an employee does make a charge of sexual harassment, the employer should investigate immediately and take appropriate action. By taking swift and decisive measures to address complaints of sexual harassment, a company signals that it takes sexual harassment seriously, thus helping reduce the likelihood of future sexual harassment.

See also: Dating Abuse; Domestic Partner Abuse; Elder Abuse; Men and Abuse; Women and Abuse; Workplace Abuse

FURTHER READING
Berman Brandenburg, Judith. *Confronting Sexual Harassment: What Schools and Colleges Can Do.* New York: Teacher's College Press, 1997.
O'Shea, Tracy, and Jane Lalonde. *Sexual Harassment: A Practical Guide to the Law, Your Rights, and Your Options for Taking Action.* New York: St. Martin's Press, 1998.
Shoop, Robert J. *Sexual Exploitation in Schools: How to Spot It and Stop It.* Thousand Oaks, CA: Corwin Press, 2003.

■ SEXUAL ASSAULT
The use of intimidation or violence to force someone to have unwanted sex. The perpetrators and victims of sexual assault include people of all ages and races. While women are most often the targets of sexual assault, men are also victims. Perhaps most distressingly, the perpetrator is most often someone the victim knows, trusts, and even loves.

INCIDENCE OF SEXUAL ASSAULT
According to the 2002 National Crime Victimization Study (NCVS), there were nearly 250,000 victims of rape or sexual assault in the United States that same year. This number included 87,000 rapes, 70,000 attempted rapes, and 91,000 sexual assaults that did not involve rape or attempted rape. Seven out of every eight victims were female. Overall, 14.8 percent of American women have been victims of rape in their lifetime. Another 2.8 percent have experienced attempted rape. By contrast, about 3 percent of men have been victims of rape or attempted rape.

Most victims of sexual assault are young, but some 20 percent are over the age of 30. Almost half (44 percent) are less than 18 years old, and 15 percent of all sexual assault victims are younger than age 12. About 80 percent of victims are white, but members of other races are victimized at higher rates than whites. According to the 1998 National Violence Against Women Survey (NVAWS), 17.7 percent of all white women reported being victims of rape or attempted rape during their lifetimes. By comparison, 18.8 percent of black women reported being victimized. The highest rates of victimization were found among Native Americans and Alaskan Natives (34.1) percent. Asians and Pacific Islanders had the lowest rate at 6.8 percent.

Contrary to a popular stereotype, sexual assault is not a crime perpetrated by strangers lurking in dark alleys. In its 1997 publication *Sex Offenses and Offenders*, the Bureau of Justice Statistics (BJS) reports that in 75.6 percent of sexual assaults, the perpetrator was a current or former partner, a relative, or a friend of the victim.

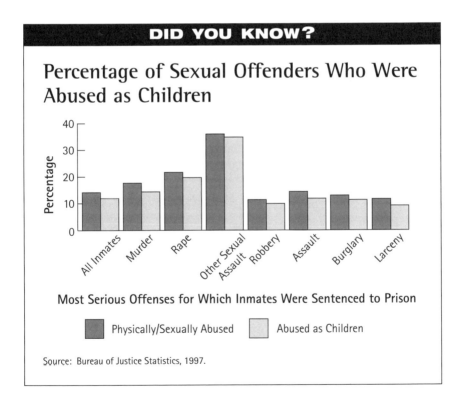

DID YOU KNOW?

Percentage of Sexual Offenders Who Were Abused as Children

Most Serious Offenses for Which Inmates Were Sentenced to Prison

Physically/Sexually Abused   Abused as Children

Source: Bureau of Justice Statistics, 1997.

According to the BJS, almost 60 percent of all sexual assaults took place in the victim's home or the home of a relative, friend, or neighbor. However, the NCVS reports that while relatives or acquaintances commit most sexual assault against women, most perpetrators of sexual assault against men are strangers to their victims.

CHARACTERISTICS OF PERPETRATORS

According to the BJS, in 1997 white males committed 73.9 percent of all sexual assaults and 52.2 percent of all rapes in the United States. Rapists and those who commit sexual assault are also older on average than other violent criminals. The BJS reports that 12 percent of sexual assaulters and 7 percent of rapists are over 50, compared to less than 5 percent of all violent offenders. The average age at arrest for all violent offenders was 29, compared to 31 for rapists and 34 for sexual assaulters.

Rapists and sexual assaulters are also more likely to have been married than other violent offenders. According to the BJS, only 47 percent of prisoners serving sentences for violent crime have ever been married. However, about 60 percent of rapists and more than 60 percent of sexual assaulters have been married.

Somewhat surprisingly, sexual offenders were less likely than other violent offenders to have a history of violence. The BJS found that 31 percent of violent offenders had prior convictions for violent crimes. About 26 percent of rapists and 25 percent of sexual assaulters had a prior conviction for violent crime. However, perpetrators of sexual assault and rape were more likely to have been victims of sexual or **physical abuse** as children. About one-third of those convicted of sexual abuse had been abused as children, compared to about 11 percent of all prison inmates. About 20 percent of rapists reported childhood sexual or physical abuse.

Fact Or Fiction?

Convicted sex offenders who are released from jail are likely to commit other sex offenses.

Fact: According to the Bureau of Justice Statistics, rapists on probation were twice as likely as other violent offenders on probation to be rearrested for rape. Released rapists were over 10 times more likely to be rearrested for rape as were those convicted of other crimes. Those released for sexual assault were 7.5 times more likely as other offenders to be rearrested for sexual assault.

RESPONDING TO SEXUAL ASSAULT

Sexual assault is a crime that should be reported immediately. The Mississippi State University Police Department, Student Health Center, and Counseling Center provide the following guidelines for victims of sexual assault:

- Go to a safe place as soon as possible.
- Preserve all physical evidence. Doing so means avoiding a bath or shower, washing one's hands, using the toilet, or changing/washing clothing before speaking to police or other law enforcement officials.
- Seek medical attention. A medical examination can not only identify any injuries suffered during the attack but also help to collect important physical evidence.
- Call the police as soon as possible.
- Seek counseling or other forms of support. Victims of sexual assault or rape need someone with whom to share their feelings after the attack.

Local rape crisis centers provide free counseling and education services about rape and sexual assault of all types. They offer 24-hour emergency hotlines, crisis intervention, individual counseling, group counseling, advocacy, accompaniment throughout the medical and/or legal process, referral, prevention education and community outreach. The centers, which began as a grassroots movement, are now important community resources that the police call whenever a rape is reported. Volunteers or staff members accompany the victims to the hospital and then through the legal proceedings. The centers provide counseling to very young victims through the use of puppets. They also help victims who have never dealt with their sexual abuse, even if it happened many years before.

Victims should be aware that the process of reporting and prosecuting a rape or sexual assault can be quite traumatic. Police and other officials will need to gather information, which means recounting and reliving the incident, possibly several times. Prosecution can be especially difficult for those assaulted by a relative or **domestic** partner. Many times the victim is reluctant to prosecute a loved one or is afraid that the perpetrator will later try to obtain revenge. Victims who are financially dependent upon their partners may hesitate to send their main source of support to jail.

Although the 2002 NCVS found that the rate of sexual assault and rape declined sharply during the previous decade, both are still significant problems for U.S. society. One of the keys to ending sexual assault is reporting the incident. Silence is not only psychologically damaging, it allows the perpetrator to continue assaulting others. Bringing sexual assault into the open is the most effective way to deal with this destructive behavior.

PREVENTING SEXUAL ASSAULT

A 2003 article by the Pennsylvania Coalition Against Domestic Violence and the National Resource Center on Domestic Violence titled "Prevention of Domestic Violence and Sexual Assault" reports that, despite increased public awareness of sexual assault, researchers are still struggling to develop effective prevention programs. According to the article, some factors that increase the likelihood that a person will commit sexual assault can be identified during childhood and adolescence. These include experiencing abuse as a child, attitudes of peers, and adolescent substance abuse. Prevention efforts need to begin at an early age to address these potential risk factors.

Prevention efforts are often categorized as primary, secondary, and tertiary. Primary efforts try to prevent sexual assault before it occurs. Secondary prevention targets people who have been identified as being at risk of committing sexual assault. Tertiary efforts try to minimize the effects of a sexual assault.

Some primary prevention efforts begin as early as elementary school. They are based on the idea that much social learning takes place at school; it is the place where the values that can prevent violent behaviors including sexual assault can be taught. Many primary prevention programs stress that students need to be aware of the problem of sexual assault and teach positive values such as personal responsibility. Others, such as programs developed by the Minnesota Coalition for Battered Women, address the root causes of violence and sexual abuse such as sexism and issues of power and control.

Primary prevention efforts aimed at adolescents often involve dispelling myths that can lead to dating violence and sexual assault. One such program was described in the 1996 book *A.S.A.P.: A School-Based Anti-violence Program.* The program relies on plays, video-tapes, and classroom discussions to encourage students to examine attitudes that might promote sexual violence. Results of a similar program were reported by a 2001 article in the *Journal of Consulting and Clinical Psychology* titled "Evaluating a Prevention Program for Teenagers on Sexual Coercion: A Differential Effectiveness Approach." The program used video presentations and an interactive "virtual date" to challenge attitudes about sexual behavior.

A number of secondary prevention programs are designed to combat rape myths and controlling behavior among adolescent males at risk for committing sexual assault, such as those raised in an abusive family atmosphere. A 1991 article in the journal *Archives of Sexual Behavior* titled "Rape Prevention with High-Risk Males: Short-term Outcome of Two Interventions," described two programs that showed promise. These programs provided information that challenged false beliefs that promoted or tolerated sexual assault, such as the idea that some women enjoy rape. The programs proved effective in changing beliefs among a high-risk group of males.

Tertiary prevention efforts for sexual assault typically take the form of counseling programs for victims, the establishment of shelters for raped and abused women, and law enforcement efforts to arrest and convict those who commit rape and sexual assault. Clearly, by the time tertiary prevention programs are needed, the victim has suffered much physical and psychological damage. Thus, it is important for local schools and communities to develop programs aimed at primary and secondary prevention. Such programs offer the greatest hope for reducing the incidence and impact of sexual assault.

See also: Abuse in Society; Child Sexual Abuse; Dating Abuse; Domestic Partner Abuse; Elder Abuse; Men and Abuse; Sexual Abuse; Women and Abuse

FURTHER READING

Giradin, Barbara W., Diana K. Faugno, Patty C. Seneski, et al. *Color Atlas of Sexual Assault.* St. Louis, MO: Mosby, 1997.
Kaminker, Laura. *Everything You Need to Know about Dealing with Sexual Assault.* New York: Rosen Publishing Group, 2002.

■ STALKING

Making unwanted contact with someone in a way that communicates a threat or causes the other person to fear for his or her safety. The word *stalking* conjures up images of a man following, spying on, and even physically assaulting a woman. However, stalking takes many different forms, and it is not a crime committed solely by men against women. According to the National Center for Violent Crime's Stalking Resource Center, stalking is a complex behavior engaged in by both sexes, and it typically indicates the presence of underlying personal or psychological problems.

INCIDENCE

Researchers compiling data on stalking face several obstacles. One is that many different activities are included under the term *stalking*. These include following and observing or telephoning someone against his or her will; collecting personal information; contacting the individual via the Internet; sending unwanted letters, notes, or gifts; and committing acts of vandalism or property damage. Another obstacle is that law enforcement agencies do not record stalking behavior as part of regular crime reports. Until recently stalking was not considered a type of criminal behavior. Stalking incidents were typically treated as cases of harassment or domestic partner abuse. In the 1980s and 1990s, however, a series of stalking incidents involving celebrities brought the issue of stalking into the public spotlight.

The largest and most current survey of stalking behavior is the 1998 National Violence Against Women Survey (NVAWS), conducted by the National Institute of Justice and the Centers for Disease Control and Prevention. This phone survey included 8,000 women and 8,000 men age 18 or older. According to the survey, about 75 percent of stalking incidents involve men stalking women. However, men make up not only 94 percent of those who stalk female victims but also 60 percent of those who stalk men. Overall, 87 percent of all stalkers are male. The study concluded that one in every 12 women will be stalked during her lifetime, compared to one in every 45 men.

Stalkers usually know their victims, often quite well. The NVAWS found that 77 percent of female victims knew their stalkers and in 59 percent of cases the stalker and victim were intimate partners. Among male victims, 64 percent knew their stalkers and 30 percent were stalked by an intimate partner. According to a 2000 study titled

"Sexual Victimization of College Women," 80.3 percent of stalking victims knew or had seen the perpetrator before the incident.

The consequences of stalking can range from fear to emotional or psychological trauma to physical and sexual assault. The NVAWS found that 45 percent of female victims felt seriously threatened by the stalker, as did 43 percent of male victims. In addition, 81 percent of the women who were stalked by a former partner were physically assaulted and 31 percent were sexually assaulted. In "Sexual Victimization of College Women," 30 percent of female victims reported emotional or

DID YOU KNOW?

Relationship of Stalkers to Their Victims

Most female stalking victims are targeted by current or former spouses, partners, or dates. Male victims are most often stalked by strangers or acquaintances.

Percentage of Cases

Relationship	Female	Male
Ex-spouse	38%	13%
Ex-partner	10%	9%
Date/Former date	14%	10%
Relative other than spouse	4%	2%
Aquaintance	19%	34%
Stranger	23%	36%

Percentage of Victims

Female (650 victims)   Male (179 victims)

Source: National Institute of Justice, 1997.

psychological trauma as a result of stalking. However, only in 15.3 percent of cases did the stalker threaten or attempt to physically assault the victim. In 10.3 percent of cases the stalker either sexually assaulted the victim or attempted to do so.

Stalking all too often results in murder. According to a 1999 article in the journal *Homicide Studies* titled "Stalking and Intimate Partner Femicide," 76 percent of all women murdered in the United States were stalked by their partners in the year before the murder. Two-thirds of these victims (67 percent) had suffered **physical abuse** from their partner in the previous 12 months. Of those female murder victims who had been physically abused, 89 percent had also been stalked in the previous year.

CHARACTERISTICS OF STALKERS

According to the National Center for Violent Crime (NCVC), most stalkers are in their 40s or younger and are above average in intelligence. Experts have identified few other traits commonly shared by stalkers. Stalkers come from all ethnic and socioeconomic backgrounds and show no single behavioral or psychological profile. Psychologists have, however, identified two general categories of stalking behavior: love obsession and simple obsession.

Love obsession occurs when a person develops a fixation on someone he or she does not personally know. This category includes people who stalk celebrities as well as those who stalk strangers or individuals with whom they have a casual relationship. For example, the victim of love obsession stalking might be a coworker or even someone seen briefly in a public place.

Love obsession stalkers usually suffer from a mental disorder. They often live in a fantasy world and create fictional relationships in which they see their victims as love interests. Stalking the victim becomes a way to act out this fantasy in the real world. The stalker also expects a victim to play along with the fantasy and may become aggressive if the victim responds negatively to the stalking behavior, which may lead to threats of violence or even physical assault and murder.

Most stalking behavior is classified as simple obsession stalking in which the victim and perpetrator share a previous relationship. This type of stalking comprises almost all incidents of stalking connected with domestic violence and dating violence. Simple obsession stalkers do not usually suffer from a mental illness, but they do have personality disorders. Such stalkers exhibit the following traits:

- Poor social skills and social adjustment
- Emotional immaturity
- Feelings of powerlessness
- Lack of success in intimate relationships
- Extreme jealousy
- Extreme insecurity

Simple obsession stalkers try to increase their self-esteem by dominating and intimidating their partners. Because the victim is the source of self-esteem, the stalker becomes fearful of losing his or her partner. If the partner leaves, the stalker may suffer a sense of worthlessness, which is what makes simple obsession stalking dangerous. At this point the stalker will do anything to regain possession of the victim. During the period immediately following the separation the target of stalking is in the greatest danger, especially if the partner has also been a victim of domestic abuse. Domestic violence victims who leave an abusive relationship are 75 percent more likely to be murdered by their partners than those who are not abused.

According to the NCVC, stalking behavior often follows certain patterns or cycles. It usually starts when the stalker makes advances toward the object of their obsession but are rejected. The stalker may at first send presents or love letters to attempt to romance the victim. When these attempts are rejected, the stalker tries to intimidate the victim by intruding into his or her life. The behavior continues until it becomes a pattern of repeated harassment, intimidation, and threatening behavior. In time the stalker, frustrated by his or her inability to control the victim, turns to violence. Unable to possess or win the love of the victim, the stalker may decide that no one else should be able to either.

Experts emphasize that although this pattern of behavior is common, stalkers are unpredictable. Some stalkers never progress past the stage of obsession and sending gifts or notes. Others jump straight from first rejection to violence and sometimes follow a violent episode by sending flowers or love letters. In other cases, long periods of time may pass between each stalking incident. The unpredictable nature of stalking behavior makes responding effectively difficult.

LAWS AGAINST STALKING

Before 1990 there were no specific state or federal laws against stalking. That year California became the first state to pass an anti-stalking law. Since that time, all 50 states as well as the federal government have passed such laws. Ten Native American nations have also passed tribal codes that define stalking and provide penalties for stalkers on tribal lands. State, tribal, and federal laws define stalking slightly differently, but all outlaw behavior aimed at harassing or threatening the safety of another person.

The federal law that addresses stalking is the 1994 Federal Interstate Stalking Law. It covers cases in which a stalker pursues a victim across state or tribal boundaries "with the intent to kill, injure, harass, or intimidate another person." It prohibits the use of mail, e-mail, and the Internet for threatening or intimidating another person. The law also protects the spouse, partner, and family members of the stalking victim. Conviction under the law is punishable by a maximum prison sentence of 20 years if the victim suffers a disfiguring or life-threatening injury. If the victim suffers "serious bodily injury" or if the offender uses a deadly weapon during the offense, the maximum sentence is 10 years. Otherwise, the maximum penalty is five years in jail. A fine may also accompany these sentences.

State statutes against stalking differ not only in their definitions of stalking but also in penalties and the kinds of actions that law enforcement authorities can take to prevent stalking. For example, some states allow police to arrest stalkers without first obtaining an warrant—a legal document that allows police to arrest an individual suspected of a crime. In other states, accused stalkers cannot be released on bail. Stalkers in some jurisdictions must undergo mandatory (legally required) psychological testing and treatment. Some states also automatically issue **restraining orders** against accused stalkers to prevent them from contacting their intended victims.

TEENS SPEAK

I Met a Really Nice Guy Last Summer—At Least He Seemed Nice at First

I went to stay with some relatives, and while my cousin and I were waiting to buy movie tickets, this cute guy came up to us. He said his name was Ron and that he had seen us at the movies before, so he decided to introduce himself.

Ron paid us both a lot of compliments and even bought us popcorn and drinks for the show. Afterward he asked me out and we dated for a few weeks. I really liked Ron, but I knew I had to go back home at the end of the summer so I didn't get too serious about him. I also told him not to get too serious about me.

About a week before I had to leave, Ron started acting kind of weird. One night I saw him hanging around my cousin's house late at night. He didn't try to come over, he just stood outside and watched the house. Then he sent me a note asking me not to go and saying we could run off together. I thought he was kidding, but the next day he came by and asked me what I thought about his idea. "What idea?" I asked. "Us running away!" he said. I told him I thought it was a joke and I started laughing. But Ron didn't laugh. He got angry and started yelling at me, telling me he wasn't going to let me go. I got scared and ran back to my cousin's house. I avoided Ron the last few days before I left.

The other day my cousin e-mailed me that Ron hung around her house for days after I left and tried to get her to tell him how to get in touch with me. I was scared that he might try to find me and come after me, because he knows which city I live in. I'm just glad it's a big town and he doesn't know my last name. Still, I'm not going to take any chances. I told my folks and some friends and teachers at school what happened, and I told them what Ron looks like. My friend Beth said I can always come to her house if I'm scared because her dad works at home and he can look out for us. I know my family and friends will keep an eye out and protect me if Ron does came around.

RESPONDING TO STALKING

Depending upon the circumstances, stalking victims may or may not be at imminent risk of danger. However, even if a victim does not feel immediately threatened by a stalker, he or she should take steps to address the issue. The NCVC has published tips and suggestions for stalking victims to help reduce the chances of being hurt by a stalker.

A person who feels in imminent danger of violence from a stalker should first find a safe place to seek protection from the stalker. This could include the home of a family member or friend (especially one whose location is unknown to the stalker); a domestic violence shelter, police station, church, or other facility that offers assistance to those in need; or busy public places where any disturbance or threat would be seen by many witnesses. A stalker may not wish to cause a scene or risk being identified while committing a violent act.

A person threatened with immediate harm should call the police as soon as he or she reaches a safe place. The victim should identify himself or herself and request that all information or records about the report be kept confidential. The victim should also report any property damage or injuries caused by the stalker. A stalking victim can receive additional help from social service agencies, victims' services agencies, and mental health professionals.

There are several options available to a victim who is fearful but does not feel immediately at risk. He or she may ask a court to issue a restraining order that requires the stalker to stay away from the victim. Violating a restraining order can result in a fine or jail time, or both. However, there is no way to ensure a stalker will obey the order, and the police cannot take action until the order is violated. By then the stalker may have had the chance to harm the victim. Some states will only issue restraining orders against current or former partners, not strangers or acquaintances. In addition, there is no guarantee that a court will grant a restraining order. A court can refuse to issue a restraining order if it feels that the perpetrator does not pose a threat to the victim.

Victims should document violations of the law committed against them or their property by stalkers. Doing so requires taking photos of damaged or vandalized property and injuries inflicted by the stalker, as well as saving notes, letters, e-mails, or messages left on telephone answering machines by the perpetrator. If these crimes are reported to the police the perpetrator can be tried under state or federal anti-stalking laws.

It is also important to have an emergency plan of action in case the threat from the stalker becomes more immediate. This should include:

- Ready access to important phone numbers, such as police and close friends;
- A list of safe locations;
- Contact numbers to call after reaching safety, such as child care, neighbors, friends, attorneys, etc.;

- A small, packed suitcase in an easy-to-locate place, such as in the trunk of the car;
- Extra cash, medications, and important documents such as passports or birth certificates; and
- If children are with the victim, a few books, toys, or other special items.

The victim should also alert police, family, friends, neighbors, and employers to the situation and enlist their aid in making a plan. Victims can take other preventive measures to increase their own safety by:

- Installing solid doors with deadbolts
- Changing locks on the house
- Installing outside lighting and trimming bushes around the house where a stalker might hide
- Getting an unlisted phone number
- Taking different routes to regular activities such as work, shopping, and dining
- Limiting the amount of time spent traveling alone, walking, or jogging
- Informing trusted neighbors, friends, and coworkers about the situation and giving them a photo of the stalker
- Giving on-site managers or security personnel at rental properties a photo of the stalker
- Screening phone calls

If you are concerned that you are being stalked, the NCVC recommends that you trust your instincts, take threats seriously, and act to ensure your safety. Don't attempt to communicate with or confront the stalker. Instead, talk to the police, the courts, and local social service agencies to obtain professional help in dealing with the problem. The law enforcement and **criminal justice system** is ready to assist victims of stalking, but they must be made aware of the problem before they can help.

See also: Dating Abuse; Domestic Partner Abuse; Sexual Abuse; Sexual Assault

FURTHER READING

Andert, Stephen. *Web Stalkers: Protect Yourself from Internet Criminals & Psychopaths.* Kitrell, NC: Rampant Tech Press, 2005.

Dunn, Jennifer. *Courting Disaster: Intimate Stalking, Culture, and Criminal Justice.* Berlin: Aldine de Gruyter, 2002.

Meloy, J. Reid. *The Psychology of Stalking: Clinical and Forensic Perspectives.* San Diego, CA: Academic Press, 2001.

Mullen, Paul E., Michelle Pathe, and Rosemary Purcell. Stalkers and Their Victims. Cambridge, UK: Cambridge University Press, 2000.

■ WOMEN AND ABUSE

Statistics from law enforcement agencies suggest that women are more often targets of abuse rather than perpetrators. *Intimate Partner Violence*, a 2000 report by the Department of Justice, stated that women were five times more likely than men to be victims of domestic violence. However, some critics have challenged the notion that women are less prone to violence than men. They argue that police statistics do not capture the full picture of women's role in abuse and point to research that shows women can be the abusers as well as the abused.

WOMEN AS VICTIMS

Government statistics reflect the view that women are victims and men are perpetrators. In 1998 the Bureau of Justice Statistic (BJS), reported that women were the victims in 876,340 cases of **domestic partner abuse** in the United States, while men were the victims in 157,330 reports. According to the BJS, domestic abuse accounts for 22 percent of all violent crime against women, and 3 percent of violent crime against men. The 2000 National Violence Against Women Survey (NVAWS) found similar numbers: 22.1 percent of the women surveyed had been physically assaulted by an intimate partner compared to 7.4 percent of male respondents.

Women are also more likely to be injured or killed as a result of domestic abuse. According to the 1992 article "Marital Aggression: Impact, Injury, and Health Correlates for Husbands and Wives," half of abused women suffer injuries from domestic violence, compared to about one-third of men. The BJS reported in 1999 that females were victims in 75 percent of the reported murders of domestic partners in the United States. The *Intimate Partner Violence* report found that one-third of all female murder victims in 2000 were killed by an intimate partner.

Females are also more likely to be victims of **child abuse** and **elder abuse**. According to a 1997 study of Child Protective Services agencies by the Department of Health and Human Services, 52 percent of child abuse victims were female. Over three-quarters (77 percent) of victims of child sexual abuse are female. Girls are also slightly more likely (51 percent to 49 percent) to be victims of **emotional abuse**. Boys were more likely to suffer from **neglect, physical abuse,** or failure to receive medical attention. According to the 2000 State Adult Protective Services Survey by the National Center on Elder Abuse, 56 percent of the victims of elder abuse in the United States are women. In about 30 percent of those cases the perpetrators are spouses, many of whom have a history of abusing their wives.

WOMEN AS PERPETRATORS

For many people, the idea of a women abusing a male partner seems improbable. They assume that because men are typically larger and physically stronger, they have little to fear from their partners. However, a significant number of studies suggest that female-to-male intimate violence is much more common than statistics indicate.

Domestic partner abuse

Before the 1970s, little research focused on the question of female-to-male domestic violence. Statistics compiled by the police and government agencies such as the Bureau of Justice indicated that men were responsible for the overwhelming majority of partner abuse. Current statistics still support that notion. For example, according to the 2001 NVAWS, women were victims of 64.4 percent of all incidents of domestic abuse in the United States, while men were victims in 35.6 percent.

However, these figures include only those incidents that are reported to police or other authorities and result in arrests. Many instances of female-to-male abuse go unreported. In addition, abusive men typically inflict much more physical damage on their partners than do abusive women. A man who is assaulted by his wife may not be injured seriously enough to seek treatment or call the police. If police officers respond to a report of domestic violence and neither party is injured, they often will not make an arrest. Also, many abused men are ashamed to report being victims of domestic abuse for fear of ridicule.

Beginning in the 1970s, some researchers turned their attention to the topic of female-to-male domestic violence. Since that time, researchers have found that the people they survey report much higher rates of abuse by women than are reflected in official statistics. For example, statistics from the Bureau of Justice show that about three female domestic partners are murdered for every murdered male partner. However, according to a 1989 study "Fatal Violence among Spouses in the United States," from 1976 to 1985 only 1.3 wives were murdered by their husbands for every murdered husband.

Other studies conducted during the same time period discovered that rates of female-to-male domestic violence may actually exceed those of male-to-female violence. According to the 1986 article "Societal Change and Change in Family Violence from 1976 to 1985 as Revealed by Two National Surveys," 11.3 percent of women reported being victims of domestic abuse compared to 12.1 percent of men. The 1990 National Family Violence Survey reported that male-to-female assault occurred in 122 of every 1,000 couples in the United States, while female-to-male assault occurred among 124 of every 1,000 couples.

Current research provides support for the idea that the level of female domestic violence is approaching or equal to that of men. In 2000 the journal *Psychological Bulletin* published a review of scholarly articles about domestic violence titled "Sex Differences in Aggression between Heterosexual Partners: A Meta-analytic Review." Based on his review of the research, the author concluded that women are more likely than men to use acts of physical aggression. In 2002 the *Journal of Interpersonal Violence* reported no difference in physical violence between men and women in dating relationships. In fact, according to the 2004 study "Adolescent Dating Violence. Do Adolescents Follow in Their Friends' or Their Parents' Footsteps?" females perpetrate dating violence slightly more often than males.

Q & A

Question: Are rates of violence among women increasing or decreasing?

Answer: Although research shows that women commit more domestic abuse than previously thought, rates of violent behavior among females are declining. According to the Bureau of Justice Statistics (BJS), rates of violent crime among women peaked in 1994 and have been falling since that time. The BJS also reported that the female murder rate has been declining since 1980. Most of the violent crime committed by women that was reported by the BJS consisted of simple assaults on other women.

Child and elder abuse

While men and women engage in domestic violence at about the same rate, women commit child abuse much more frequently than men. According to the Department of Health and Human Services' Administration for Children, Youth, and Families (ACF) the victim's mother acting alone perpetrated 40.3 percent of all cases of child abuse in 2002. Overall, women were responsible for 62.3 percent of all cases of child abuse. They were much more likely to neglect a child than men—73.9 percent of all cases of child neglect reported by ACF were perpetrated by women. By contrast, the ACF reports that females are much less likely to sexually abuse children. Although women committed more child abuse overall, men were responsible for 74.1 percent of all cases of child sexual abuse. The ACF found that neither sex was more likely than the other to engage in physical abuse or psychological abuse of children.

Statistics show that men and women commit elder abuse at similar rates. The National Center on Elder Abuse found that women committed 48.9 percent of all cases of elder abuse in the United States in 1996, while men committed 47.4 percent. In the remaining 3.7 percent, the sex of the perpetrator was unknown or unreported. Other studies have found that males commit most elder abuse. For example, the 2000 State Adult Protective Services Survey reported that 52 percent of the identified perpetrators of elder abuse were men. Most cases of sexual abuse of elders, however, are committed by men.

Fact Or Fiction?

Women who commit abuse are trying to be like men.

Fact: Women who commit abuse share many characteristics with abusive men, but they are not trying to be men. Although men are socialized to be aggressive, all people are capable of violence under certain circumstances. Like men, women use physical or emotional violence to gain power and control over their victims. Like many male batterers, female batterers witnessed violence at home and learned that it was the way to communicate.

Factors contributing to abuse

Researchers have proposed several theories to explain the causes of violence by females. According to a 1998 review of studies published in the *American Journal of Drug and Alcohol Abuse*, most of these theories indicate that factors other than gender determine who will become abusive. The article, "Women, Violence with Intimates, and Substance Abuse: Relevant Theory, Empirical Findings, and Recommendations for Future Research," cites research from the United States as well as other nations that shows similar rates of violence for both sexes.

The article identified two factors that seemed to increase the likelihood of abuse among females: substance abuse and a history of abuse as a child. Alcohol abuse was found to be a significant factor in the increasing use of physical violence against both spouses and children. According to a 1991 study "Substance Abuse and Serious Child Maltreatment: Prevalence, Risk, and Outcome in a Court Sample," almost half of the abusive parents surveyed had substance abuse problems. Alcohol and **cocaine** were the two drugs most frequently abused by respondents.

A 1989 article in the journal *Developmental Psychopathology* titled "Family Deviance and Family Disruption in Childhood: Associations with Maternal Behavior and Infant Maltreatment during the First Two Years of Life," reported that women who had been abused as children were more likely to abuse their own children. Other studies have drawn a connection between domestic violence and child abuse. In the 1994 study "Linking Marital Violence, Mother-Child/Father-Child Aggression, and Child Behavior Problems," 90 percent of the women surveyed in battered women's shelters displayed aggressive behavior toward their children.

With so much evidence indicating little difference in the rates of violent behavior between men and women, why are men still seen as the main perpetrators of abuse? Denise Hien, the author of *Women, Violence with Intimates, and Substance Abuse: Relevant Theory, Empirical Findings, and Recommendations for Future Research,* argues that some researchers may be reluctant to undertake or publish research suggesting that women may be as violent as men. For example, Suzanne Steinmetz wrote *The Battered Husband Syndrome* in 1977. It was one of the first in-depth examinations of female-on-male violence. Colleagues who disagreed with Steinmetz's conclusions accused her of twisting her research results to fit her theory.

Hien also points out that many of the studies of female violence indicate that poor and minority women make up most of the perpetrators of female violence. She suggests that some researchers are reluctant to publish studies that seem to blame a group of people widely perceived as victims. Whatever the reasons, the role of females as perpetrators of abuse is still largely unrecognized and underappreciated.

See also: Abuse in Society; Child Abuse; Child Sexual Abuse; Dating Abuse; Domestic Partner Abuse; Elder Abuse; Men and Abuse

FURTHER READING
Carter, Jay. *Nasty Women.* New York: McGraw-Hill, 2003.
Pearson, Patricia. *When She Was Bad: How and Why Women Get Away with Murder.* New York: Penguin Books, 1998.
Renzetti, Claire M., Jeffrey L. Edelson, and Raquel Kennedy Bergen. *Sourcebook on Violence against Women.* Thousand Oaks, CA: Sage Publications, 2000.

■ WORKPLACE ABUSE

The use of power or sexual behavior on the job to intimidate or control a coworker or employee. Every day, large numbers of workers in the United States suffer bullying, **verbal abuse,** and **sexual harassment** at the workplace. Not only do these behaviors take a physical and psychological toll on their victims, but they also cost businesses millions of dollars in lost productivity and legal costs associated with discrimination and harassment lawsuits. In recent years employers and the federal government have increased significantly their efforts to prevent workplace abuse.

SEXUAL HARASSMENT AT WORK

Perhaps the most well-known and widely publicized form of workplace abuse is **sexual harassment**–persistent and unwelcome acts or comments of a sexual nature. Sexual harassment takes two forms: quid pro quo and hostile environment. In quid pro quo harassment, a person offers someone either favors in return for sex or threatens some type of harm if the person refuses to have sex. For example, a manager who promises to promote a subordinate in exchange for sex is engaging in quid pro quo harassment. Quid pro quo harassment also occurs when a manager threatens to fire or deny a promotion to an employee who refuses to have sex.

Sexual harassment does not always involve requests or demands for sex. It can also consist of unwelcome sexual advances, physical touching of a sexual nature, demeaning or degrading sexual comments, and other acts such as posting pornography in a public workspace or telling jokes of a sexual nature. A hostile environment is created when such behavior is so frequent and intimidating that a person feels threatened or is unable to perform his or her job properly. In order to qualify as a hostile environment, the sexual comments or behaviors must be unwanted and persistent. Behavior such as telling off-color jokes at work or flirting with coworkers is not considered harassment if no one objects to or is offended by it.

TEENS SPEAK

I Am Being Harassed by the Girls I Work With

They whistle at me, send me notes, and make sexual remarks about me. At first I was flattered, but now I am getting frustrated and angry about it. They seem to show up wherever I go—sometimes they even hang around outside the restroom when I'm in there. I've called in sick a few times because I just didn't think I could deal with their "attention." They don't do anything real sexual, other than the whistling and making comments about my body.

I have asked them to leave me alone, but they don't get it. Now they whisper and laugh when I walk by, and it is making me paranoid.

I know that this isn't something that guys usually complain about. It is humiliating. I told my Dad, but he laughed and said I was lucky the girls notice me. But I don't feel so lucky. I'm afraid to tell my supervisor because she's made some comments too, and I know she won't do anything about it. Now I understand how girls feel when guys stare at them. I don't think I feel as scared as a girl might because I don't worry about them raping me or anything like that, but it's affecting my job performance. I think a lot about quitting, but I need the money, so I don't really know what to do. It is all really humiliating.

Incidence of harassment

Sexual harassment is a violation of Title VII of the Civil Rights Act of 1964, but the first sexual harassment case under that law was not decided until 1976. That year a poll published by *Redbook* magazine found that 90 percent of women surveyed had been the target of unwanted sexual advances at work. Four years later a survey of federal government employees discovered that 42 percent of women and 15 percent of men had experienced sexual harassment on the job.

More recent studies have confirmed the fact that sexual harassment on the job is a significant problem. In a 1994 telephone poll by Lou Harris and Associates, 31 percent of female respondents reported they had been sexually harassed at work. In every case, the harasser was a man. Women were more likely to be harassed by a supervisor (43 percent of all cases) than workers at the same or lower level of authority. Another 27 percent were harassed by senior employees who were not their supervisors. In 19 percent of the cases, the perpetrator was a coworker at the same level as the victim. Eight percent of female victims were harassed by a junior employee. The Harris Poll also found that 7 percent of male employees have suffered harassment. The perpetrator in 59 percent of those cases was female.

Costs of harassment

Sexual harassment on the job takes a toll on both victims and the workplace where it occurs. According to the counseling center at the University of Oregon, victims of sexual harassment may suffer a variety of psychological and physical problems, including:

- Depression
- Anxiety, fear, shock, and denial
- Anger, frustration, and irritability
- Insecurity, embarrassment, and feelings of betrayal
- Confusion and feelings of powerlessness
- Shame, guilt, and self-blame
- Low self-esteem
- Headaches
- Tiredness, listlessness, or lack of energy
- Stomach and intestinal problems

- Skin reactions such as rashes or acne
- Weight changes
- Sleep disturbances and nightmares
- Panic reactions and phobias (irrational fears)
- Sexual problems

Sexual harassment can seriously affect productivity, work performance, attendance, and job stability. In 1990 *Working Woman* magazine conducted a survey of the costs of sexual harassment at 160 corporations employing some 3.3 million workers. The survey found that sexual harassment costs the typical Fortune 500 company $6.7 million per year in absenteeism, low productivity, and employee turnover. These figures do not include legal costs for harassment lawsuits or damage done to the company's image that could result in lost business. More recent research done by prominent sexual harassment researcher and consultant Freada Klein has shown similar results.

One measure of the legal costs of sexual harassment comes from data compiled by the federal government's Equal Employment Opportunity Commission (EEOC). Since 1992 the EEOC has gathered statistics on the number of sexual harassment suits filed and resolved under Title VII. In 2003, 13,533 sexual harassment cases were filed under Title VII. Of those, 85.3 percent were filed by women. Companies involved in these suits paid out a total of $50 million in benefits to the victims of sexual harassment.

DID YOU KNOW?

Sexual Harassment Charges Settled by EEOC, 1997–2003

	1997	1998	1999	2000	2001	2002	2003
Number of Cases	15,889	15,618	15,222	15,836	15,475	14,396	13,566
Amount Paid	$49.5	$34.3	$50.3	$54.6	$53.0	$50.3	$50.0

(Note: Amounts paid are in millions of dollars)

Source: Equal Employment Opportunity Commission, 2003.

Responding to workplace harassment

Because sexual harassment on the job is so widespread and because it is a federal offense, the EEOC urges employers to take steps to create a positive work environment and respond quickly to charges of sexual harassment. There are several ways in which a company can address the issue of sexual harassment before it occurs. Every company should have a written policy on sexual harassment that clearly spells out the types of behavior that will not be tolerated. The policy should also explain penalties for violations, provide a detailed description of procedures for filing complaints, and provide a list of additional resources or contact persons employees can consult in case of harassment.

Of course, simply having a policy does not guarantee that sexual harassment will not occur in a workplace. Employers must enforce the policy consistently and aggressively, following up any charge of harassment. They must also make sure managers are aware of the policy and follow it. Under federal law, an employer is responsible for acts of harassment committed by managers or supervisors. Top executives cannot avoid responsibility by claiming they were not aware of the actions of managers who report to them. These rules also apply to third parties who work for a company on a contract basis.

All investigations should be conducted swiftly and in a way that protects the rights of both the accuser and the accused, which means that the charges must be kept confidential. In addition, someone other than a direct supervisor—such as a personnel officer—should be the person responsible for handling complaints about harassment to ensure that an employee who is being harassed by a supervisor can report the incident to a neutral party. If the complaint is upheld, the perpetrator will be punished according to the company's policy on sexual harassment. The company's failure to deal effectively with sexual harassment at the workplace can lead to expensive legal action.

Q & A

Question: What legal steps can I take if I am sexually harassed on the job?

Answer: Under Title VII, a victim of workplace sexual harassment can collect back pay and lost wages suffered due to harassment and can recover his or her job if fired. In 1991, however, the federal government amended the Civil Rights Act of 1991 to allow victims of sexual harassment to collect damages for emotional pain and suffering, mental anguish, inconvenience, and loss of enjoyment of life. An employer may also be assessed punitive damages if the victim can show that the employer acted maliciously or was indifferent to the harassment. The total amount of damages one can collect ranges from $50,000 to $300,000, depending upon the size of the company.

WORKPLACE BULLYING

Although not as widespread as workplace sexual harassment, bullying is still a significant problem for many businesses. The Workforce Bullying and Trauma Institute (WBTI) defines bullying as "repeated illegitimate mistreatment of a targeted employee by one or more persons characterized by acts of commission and omission which impair the target's psychological and physical health and economic security." Bullying can take many forms, including:

- Physical aggression
- Verbal abuse such as screaming, yelling, or publicly humiliating an employee or coworker
- Constantly criticizing or belittling an employee, tearing down an employee's confidence, or placing excessive emphasis on unimportant details of the job
- Controlling resources to prevent an employee from successfully completing projects
- Gossiping about an employee, manipulating others' impression of a coworker, or criticizing an employee to superiors or upper management

Incidence of workplace bullying

The best estimates of the incidence and nature of workplace bullying come from two studies. A study by Wayne State University in 2000 estimated that 16.8 percent of American workers experience bullying in the workplace. That same year the WBTI conducted the largest research project on workplace bullying, the U.S. Hostile Workplace Study. The study surveyed 1,335 people from across the United States who were victims of workplace bullying. It provides a snapshot of who bullies, who is bullied, and the effects of such behavior.

The study found that bullying is evenly split between men and women—half of all bullies are women and half are men. However, most of the victims (77 percent) were women. In most cases, women were targeted by other women. About 84 percent of female victims said they experienced bullying from women; 69 percent said they were bullied by men (clearly some female victims were bullied by both women and men). Although victimized less often, men endured bullying for longer periods of time. The average duration of bullying for male victims was 18.38 months compared to 15.74 months for female victims.

Most bullies were in positions of power or authority over their victims. The survey found that 81 percent of bullies were at least one level of management above their victims. One in seven bullies (14 percent) were of the same rank as the victim, while only 5 percent of bullies targeted employees in superior positions. While many observers believe that most victims are uneducated or unskilled, the data shows otherwise. The survey found that 84 percent of victims had either some college experience, an undergraduate degree, or an advanced degree. Only one in six victims had a high school education or less.

The U.S. Hostile Workplace Study also asked respondents what caused the bullying they experienced. In 58 percent of the cases, victims said they were targeted because they resisted being controlled or dominated by the perpetrator. Over half of the victims also felt that the bully envied their competence at the job. Other frequently mentioned reasons for bullying included envy of the victim's popularity or social skills (49 percent), retaliation against the victim for reporting unethical conduct by the perpetrator (46 percent), and the fact that the bully had a "cruel personality" (42 percent). However, 36 percent of victims said the bullying was unprovoked.

Fact Or Fiction?

Workplace bullies typically pick on minorities or members of other groups who are often discriminated against on the job.

Fact: According to the U.S. Hostile Workplace Survey, 38 percent of the victims of workplace bullying are not members of a so-called protected group based on gender, race, ethnicity, religion, age or disability. Members of such groups who suffer bullying can file discrimination lawsuits based on their protected status. However, because the majority of victims are not members of protected groups, they have no legal remedy unless they can prove that the bullying threatens their health or safety.

Costs of workplace bullying

As with sexual harassment, bullying can cause significant psychological and physical trauma to the victim, as well as increased costs for the business where it occurs. The U.S. Hostile Workplace Study included a health checklist to assess the effects of bullying on victims. The list below of symptoms reported by at least half of the victims is followed by the percentage who reported experiencing that symptom:

- Severe anxiety (94)
- Sleep disruption (84)
- Loss of concentration (82)
- Nervousness or edginess (80)
- Constantly thinking about the bullying (76)
- Stress headaches (64)

Other frequently reported psychological symptoms include shame, recurrent memories of abuse, **depression**, substance abuse, and panic attacks. Many victims also suffered physical complaints such as racing heartbeat, exhaustion, body aches, jaw tightening, teeth grinding, chronic (long-term) fatigue, intestinal distress, migraine headaches, and chest pains.

According to an article in the March 18, 2002 edition of the *Orlando Business Journal,* workplace bullying costs U.S. businesses more than $180 million in lost time and productivity. These costs include absenteeism, reduced productivity, stress-related illnesses, and high turnover. The U.S. Hostile Workplace Study found that 82 percent of people targeted by a bully left their workplace. Of those, 38 percent left voluntarily while 44 percent were fired or laid off. Over half of the victims surveyed lost income as a result of bullying, usually due to termination following the bullying. However, 33 percent of all targets of bullying reported no change in income. In addition, 16 percent of victims actually increased their income as a result of leaving the abusive workplace and finding a higher-paying job elsewhere.

Responding to workplace bullying

Unlike sexual harassment, most behaviors related to workplace bullying are not illegal. Thus, a victim whose employer does nothing to prevent bullying often has few options except tolerating the abuse or leaving the job. To make matters worse, many complaints of workplace bullying are ignored or not taken seriously. According to the U.S. Hostile Workplace Study, 40 percent of those who filed bullying complaints with their bosses said the boss took no action. Even worse, 42 percent of the time the boss reacted negatively to the complaint. Only 18 percent of the time did the employee's boss take positive steps to end the bullying. Human resource departments were no better at dealing with charges of bullying. In 51 percent of the cases reported to human resources personnel, no action was taken, and negative actions were taken 32 percent of the time. In only 7 percent of reported cases of bullying was the perpetrator disciplined by reprimand, transfer, or termination.

Psychologist Michael Harrison, who consults with companies about issues of workplace abuse, recommends that the victim tell the perpetrator that his or her actions are unacceptable. Ideally, the warning should be written and a copy of the note should also be sent to the company's president or human resources department. If these steps do not stop the bullying, the employee should contact a lawyer of the U.S. Department of Labor to determine whether he or she can seek legal remedies. Occupational Safety and Health Administration regulations require employers to provide a safe and healthy workplace. Victims can take their employers to court if they can show that the bullying constitutes a workplace hazard.

However, as the U.S. Hostile Workplace Study showed, in many cases the only way to end the bullying was to leave the workplace where it occurred. This can be a traumatic and financially difficult move but one that may be necessary. Respondents to the study said that recovering from the effects of workplace bullying was made easier by self-determination, emotional strength, deciding to fight back, support from family and friends, and personal faith. Given its personal and financial costs, it appears that employers need to do more to positively address and prevent workplace bullying.

See also; Men and Abuse; Sexual Abuse; Sexual Assault; Women and Abuse

FURTHER READING

Davenport, Noa, Ruth D. Schwarz, and Gail Pursell Elliott. *Mobbing: Emotional Abuse in the American Workplace, 2002.* New York: Civil Society Publishing, 2002.

Gregory, Raymond F. *Unwelcome and Unlawful: Sexual Harassment in the American Workplace.* Ithaca, NY: ILR Press, 2002.

Hornstein, Harvey A. *The Haves and the Have Nots: The Abuse of Power and Privilege in the Workplace ... and How to Control It.* London: Financial Times/Prentice Hall, 2002.

Naime, Gary, and Ruth Naime. *The Bully at Work: What You Can Do to Stop the Hurt and Reclaim Your Dignity on the Job.* Naperville, IL: Sourcebooks, 2000.

Webb, Susan L. *Step Forward: Sexual Harassment in the Workplace: What You Need to Know!* Master Media Publishing, 1997.

HOTLINES
AND HELP SITES

Bully OnLine
URL: http://www.bullyonline.org
Program: Provides online information, research, and statistics on bullying at school, in the workplace, and in the family

Childhelp National Child Abuse Hotline/Voices for Children
Phone: 1-800-4ACHILD or 1-800-422-4453; 1-800-2A-CHILD (TDD)
(24 hours a day, 7 days a week)
Program: Provides multilingual crisis intervention and counseling on child abuse; gives referrals to local social service groups offering child abuse counseling; provides literature on child abuse in English and Spanish

Girls and Boys Town National Hotline
URL: http://www.girlsandboystown.org/hotline
Phone: 1-800-448-3000; 1-800-448-1833 (TDD) (24 hours a day, 7 days a week)
Affiliation: Boys Town children's home and shelter
Program: Provides counseling for families dealing with physical and sexual abuse of children

National Center for Elder Abuse
URL: http://www.elderabusecenter.org
Phone: 1-800-677-1116 (National Eldercare Locator hotline provides contact information for state hotlines 24 hours a day, 7 days a week)
Affiliation: National Association of State Units on Aging

Program: Provides information, education, and training on dealing with and preventing elder abuse; advises lawmakers on issues of elder abuse

Mission: To promote understanding, sharing of knowledge, and action on elder abuse, neglect, and exploitation

National Coalition Against Domestic Violence

URL: http://www.ncavd.org

Phone: 1-800-799-7233 (24 hours a day, 7 days a week)

Program: Organizes and supports programs and shelters for battered women and their children and works to pass laws to end discrimination and other misuses of power that the group believes create the conditions that lead to abuse

Mission: To work for major societal changes necessary to eliminate both personal and societal violence against women and children

National Youth Violence Prevention Resource Center

URL: http://www.safeyouth.org

Phone: 1-866-SAFEYOUTH

Affiliation: Centers for Disease Control and Prevention

Program: Provides information and resources to help resolve conflicts nonviolently, stop bullying, prevent teen suicide, and end violence committed by and against young people

Project D.A.T.E.

URL: http://www.projectdate.org

Program: Provides online information about dating abuse and how to prevent it

Mission: To educate high school students about dating abuse through the Internet, pamphlets, and community and classroom presentations

Rape, Abuse, and Incest Network National Center

URL: http://www.rainn.org

Phone: 1-800-656-HOPE (24 hours a day, 7 days a week)

Program: Provides counseling for victims of rape and sexual abuse; educates the public about sexual assault; works to improve support services available to victims of sexual assault and ensure that perpetrators are brought to justice

SAFE Self-mutilation Hotline
Phone: 1-800-DONT-CUT (24 hours a day, 7 days a week)
Program: Provides counseling and advice for teens struggling with self-mutilation

Stalking Resource Center
URL: http://www.ncvc.org.src
Phone: 1-800-FYI-CALL (24 hours a day, 7 days a week)
Affiliation: National Center for Victims of Crime
Program: Provides victim assistance as well as information and training for local social welfare and law enforcement agencies about dealing with and preventing stalking
Mission: To raise national awareness of stalking and to encourage the development of multidisciplinary responses to stalking in local communities

stophazing.org
URL: http://www.stophazing.org
Program: Provides up-to-date hazing information for students, parents, and educators
Mission: To eliminate hazing through education

The Workplace Bullying and Trauma Institute
URL: http://www.bullyinginstitute.org
Phone: 1-360-656-6630 (8 A.M.–6 P.M. PST, M-F)
Program: Provides information about workplace bullying to employees and employers; sponsors research into and conferences about workplace bullying; offers training to help employers identify and eliminate workplace bullying
Mission: To raise societal awareness of and create solutions for workplace bullying

GLOSSARY

AIDS (acquired immune deficiency syndrome) a chronic disease caused by the human immunodeficiency virus (HIV) in which the immune system is weakened and unable to fight infections

amphetamines a class of mood-changing drugs often used illegally; taken together with alcohol, they can cause severe stomach distress, keep drinkers awake, and lead to dangerous overdoses of alcohol

barbiturates prescription drugs that depress the central nervous system; used to treat anxiety, tension, and sleep disorders

battered an individual who is frequently abused

batterer someone who frequently abuses others

battering frequent and repeated abuse

caregiver someone responsible for the welfare of another person, particularly a child or elderly person

cocaine illicit drug derived from the coca plant that increases energy and alertness and elevates self-confidence

corporal punishment physical punishment, such as beating or spanking

criminal justice system   institutions that enforce the law and punish those who violate the law; includes police, prosecutors, judges, jails, prisons, probation boards, and parole boards

date rape drug   a drug administered without the user's consent that causes unconsciousness and makes the victim helpless against sexual assault

dependent   someone who relies on another person to take care of his or her basic needs

depressants   drugs that lower the level of mental and physical activity

depression   a mental condition marked by feelings of extreme sadness or worthlessness and often thoughts of suicide

domestic partner   a spouse or person with whom one lives and shares a long-term sexual relationship

emotional abuse   an attempt to control a person by withholding affection or attention or by manipulating his or her emotions

felony   a serious crime punishable by a sentence in a state or federal prison

financial abuse   an attempt to control someone by withholding or denying financial support

heredity   the passing of traits from parent to child

heroin   an illicit drug derived from the Asian poppy that causes drowsiness, relieves pain, and produces euphoria

HIV (human immunodeficiency virus)   the organism that causes AIDS (acquired immune deficiency syndrome)

infanticide   the killing of an unwanted baby

juvenile   legal term for a person under the age of 18

learned helplessness condition in which a victim exposed to repeated trauma or punishment stops trying to escape

mandated legally required

marijuana an illicit drug derived from the plant *Cannabis sativa* that produces relaxation, alters mood, and distorts the way the user experiences sights, sounds, or other senses

methamphetamines nervous system stimulants that are related to amphetamines, which have similar but much more intense effects

misdemeanor a crime punishable by a fine and/or a sentence in a local or county jail

neglect failure to care for the physical or emotional needs of a dependent person

neurotransmitter a chemical that allows nerve cells to communicate with one another to maintain normal physical and psychological functioning

paranoia extreme and unreasonable feelings of persecution

parole the early release of a person from prison as long as all conditions of the release are met

PCP (phencyclidine) powerful illicit central nervous system depressant originally used as an anesthetic; also known as "angel dust"

patriarchal marked by male domination and control of power

peer an individual of one's own age and/or economic or social status

physical abuse the use of strength, weapons, or the threat of injury to hurt or control another person

probation a sentencing alternative by a court by which convicted defendants are released on suspended sentences, generally under the supervision of a probation officer as long as certain conditions are observed

restraining order   an document issued by a court that orders an abuser to stay away from his or her intended victim

schizophrenia   a mental disorder marked by loss of touch with reality

sexual exploitation   the use of a position of power or authority to coerce someone to have sex

sexually transmitted diseases (STDs)   a disease that can be passed from one person to another during sexual relations

steroids   drugs used to increase muscle mass and strength

stimulant   a drug that improves alertness, reduces fatigue, and elevates mood

support group   a group of people at various stages of recovery from abuse who offer one another support, assistance, and advice

verbal abuse   the use of yelling, name-calling, and insults to intimidate, humiliate, or control another person

victim advocate   person who helps victims of abuse understand and deal with the legal process of prosecuting offenders

INDEX

Page numbers in *italic* indicate graphs or sidebars. Page numbers in **bold** represent extensive coverage of a topic.